Comments on *Kidney Failure Explained* from readers

'This book is, without doubt, the best resource currently available for kidney patients and those who care for them.'
Val Said, Kidney transplant patient

'*Kidney Failure Explained* not only answered all the questions I wanted to ask, it also answered a lot of questions I hadn't even thought of. Books of this kind are badly needed. Thank you for a clear and precise text, in language I can understand.'
Dennis Jackson, CAPD patient

'Your book has been a tremendous help and support throughout. I think that *Kidney Failure Explained* should be offered to all renal patients.'
J. R., Kidney donor, Northampton 'I was so impressed by the wonderful way the book is presented, in terms which everyone can understand. Our committee has recommended the book to our members.'
Roy Bradbury, Chairman, Sheffield Area Kidney Association

'This is a very well written book and it should be of great value to renal patients.'
Professor R. Wilkinson, Consultant Nephrologist, Freeman Group of Hospitals, Newcastle-upon-Tyne

'The book is excellent and will prove very valuable to a variety of different groups. I shall certainly be recommending it to patients and to general practitioners in particular.'
Dr Robin Winney, Consultant Renal Physician, Department of Renal Medicine, The Royal Infirmary of Edinburgh

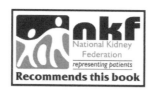

Recommends this book

The National Kidney Federation (NKF) is a charity representing all kidney patients in the United Kingdom, it is run by Kidney patients for Kidney patients. The Federation campaigns for increased renal provision and improved treatment. The charity also provides national services to assist all kidney patients.

Publications recommended by the NKF have to be of a high standard and easily readable, the recommendation is not given lightly and is highly prized. The NKF recommendation of this book was made at the time of its publication and has to be renewed at subsequent prints in order to retain the NKF endorsement and recommendation. Further information about the NKF and books it recommends can be found on its website www.kidney.org.uk.

KIDNEY FAILURE EXPLAINED

Everything you always wanted to know about
dialysis and kidney transplants
but were afraid to ask

Dr Andy Stein, MD, FRCP

Consultant Nephrologist and Acute Physician, University Hospitals,
Coventry and Warwickshire NHS Trust

Janet Wild, RGN

Clinical Education Manager, Baxter Healthcare Ltd, Newbury, Berkshire

CLASS PUBLISHING • LONDON

Class Health, Barb House, Barb Mews, London W6 7PA, UK
Email: Post@Class.co.uk
Website www.Class.co.uk

Class Health is an imprint of Class Publishing Ltd, a company registered in England No. 2993127. VAT No: GB 503 5208 87
Registered Office: 7 Melrose Terrace, London W6 7RL, UK

Printing history
First published 1999
Reprinted with revisions 2000
Second edition 2002
Third edition 2007
Fourth edition 2010

A CIP Catalogue for this book is available from the British Library

10 9 8 7 6 5 4 3 2 1

ISBN 978 1 85959 236 6

Edited by Richenda Milton-Daws

Designed and illustrated by Darren Bennett

Typeset by Typematter, Basingstoke

Printed and bound in Slovenia by arrangement with KINT, Ljubljana

CONTENTS

FOREWORD

If ever proof were required that this book is desperately needed, look no further than the National Kidney Federation telephone Helpline. That Helpline takes more than 200 calls per week from concerned kidney patients, nearly all of whom would have found the answer to their worries in this book. This is why the book is the most sort after by kidney patients, and it is why this book is the most popular that the NKF recommends. It has been the most popular book since the first edition was published in 1999.

Kidney failure is indeed complex; little wonder then that raising the profile of kidney disease amongst the public is so hard. Raising the profile is necessary to ensure that kidney patients get the treatment and resources they deserve, and that opinion formers are fully aware of the everyday plight of kidney patients. This book, so clear and so comprehensive, helps to inform and to educate. It is a real boon in the NKF's armory for a fairer deal for our patient members.

Kidney disease, together with its treatment, is changing all the time – and very quickly. That is a good thing, for there is much more to be done, more to be found out, and more work necessary to improve patients' quality of life and life expectancy. Andy Stein and Janet Wild have realised this; that is why they have written a new edition. Patients need to realise it too. Even if, like your fellow patients, you purchased an earlier copy, it's time to upgrade, time to re-learn, time to re-evaluate your condition and your treatment, and time to ensure you are doing the very best for yourself. This book tells you.

Timothy F Statham OBE
Chief Executive
National Kidney Federation

FOREWORD

I am delighted to be able to write a Foreword to this fourth Edition of *Kidney Failure Explained*. The authors, Andy Stein and Janet Wild, continue to improve the book with each edition, ensuring it is brought right up to date, with information about many recent developments in kidney care.

This remains simply the best book of its kind; the book I recommend to people I meet who have just found out they have serious kidney disease, and are confronted by so much uncertainty, so much new information, and so many decisions that they do not know where to start. This book packs in a remarkable amount of practical information as well as some complex ideas, always explains things clearly and simply without ever patronising.

Because it is such a helpful book for people with kidney disease to read, it is of course also very important that all doctors, and other health professionals involved in caring for kidney patients, read it. It will help them with the first and most important art – to communicate with people on their terms, and so help to give them new confidence to keep control of their lives despite all that is happening to them.

John Feehally
Professor of Renal Medicine
Leicester

ACKNOWLEDGEMENTS

Kidney disease is about teamwork. This book could not have been written without the combined efforts of the following people. Professor Gerry Coles (Cardiff) inspired Andy Stein to be a kidney doctor, for which he is thanked. He was subsequently inspired by Dwomoa Adu (QE Birmingham), Tim Mathew (Adelaide, Australia), the late Professor John Walls (Leicester) and Hugh Cairns (King's, London). He has many brilliant current colleagues, especially Rob Higgins, Simon Fletcher and Mair Edmunds, with whom he is honoured to work. John Walls's favourite phrase 'Just Do It' summarises his approach to medicine.

Early in Janet Wild's renal career, she met many enthusiastic people, with most of whom she is still privileged to work. Amongst these are, of course, her co-author and friend Andy Stein whose outlook and attitude to life have made writing so much fun. Donna Lamping, Jean Hooper and Claire Bradley are three psychologists who individually highlighted the importance of good, clear communication and education to Janet. Carina Nilsson, a colleague from Baxter, has continued to coach and inspire her over the years. Ram Gokal, Simon Davies, Edwina Brown and Martin Wilkie are nephrologists who continue to teach, encourage and motivate not only Janet but many other healthcare professionals they meet.

John Walls and Professor Terry Feest (Bristol) were the first doctors to review the first edition of the book, and both devoted much time to improving it. Subsequently the book was also reviewed by Dr Gillian Matthews (Andy's mother), Dr Steve Nelson (St George's, London), Dr Rob Higgins (Coventry) and Dr Phin Kon (King's, London). The guest writers, Juliet Auer (Oxford), Gemma Bircher (Leicester), Peter Ellis (King's, London), Jean Hooper (Gloucester), Dr Ian Lawrence (Leicester) and Althea Mahon (Royal London Hospital) all took to their task keenly and with speed. Individual chapters were reviewed by Mr Mark Emberton (UCL), Mr Paul Gibbs (King's, London), Professor John Cunningham (UCL), Professor Mike Nicholson (Leicester), Dr Ian Abbs (Guy's, London), Mr Geoff Koffman (Guy's, London) and Dr Roger Greenwood (Stevenage). For this edition, we are particularly grateful to Professor John Feehally and Tim Statham OBE for writing such encouraging Forewords.

The early force behind the book was Val Said, a kidney patient, who works tirelessly as a volunteer advocate for patients with kidney failure in the UK. Her efforts have been subsequently supported by Austin Donohoe, formerly Chairman of the National Kidney Federation.

The publisher, Richard Warner, insisted on literary excellence but never 'pushed' us faster than we could cope with. Darren Bennett is (again) thanked for his clear diagrams and design, and Judith Wise for her tireless work in marketing the book. We also thank Ruth Midgley and Richenda Milton-Daws, editors of the four editions, for insisting on factual accuracy and clear writing for our readers. They converted this book from something that was 'alright' to something about which we are proud.

This list would not be complete without our thanking our families for supporting us, in particular our partners Emma and Chris.

Andy Stein and Janet Wild

INTRODUCTION

This is a book about kidney failure and its treatment. It is rare that kidney failure affects only the person who has been given the diagnosis. It affects whole families, friends and work colleagues. The diagnosis can be as devastating for those on the sidelines as it is for the person at the centre. But, for many people, finding out information and learning to understand their illness can help them get to grips with the problems. With this in mind we have written a book that we hope will be useful to anyone affected by kidney failure.

Both authors of this book believe that the more you know about your kidney failure and its treatment, the better you will be able to cope with it. Kidney medicine, along with all medical specialties, is rife with jargon, abbreviations and acronyms. However, once you get through all the specialist terminology, there should be no aspect of healthcare that is too complicated or difficult to explain. In this book, we have set out to dispel the myths, unravel the jargon and explain all matters of the kidney as simply and straightforwardly as possible.

The aim therefore is to give you, the reader, the knowledge and confidence to ask questions. This in turn will make it easier for you to get the right information, phrased in the right way. Then you can use this information to make the choices that are best for you, take control of what happens to you and enjoy your life in spite of your kidney failure.

As with many other areas of medicine, there are controversies and differences of opinion in the treatment of kidney failure. We have tried hard to represent the views of the majority and to explain why these disagreements exist.

We've also included some details of the politics that surround the treatment of kidney failure; including the disparities between areas of the UK, and around the world. For example there is a wide variation in the number of patients who receive a kidney from a living donor, or who are offered the choice to do their dialysis at home. Access to home haemodialysis and peritoneal dialysis is not equal around the UK, and there are differences in transplant success rates.

It's more than 10 years since we wrote the first edition of this book. We've tried hard to keep it up to date and relevant to all our readers during that time. Although a lot has changed since the days before ESAs, when dialysis was denied to older people, and access to APD and living donor transplantation was very limited, a diagnosis of kidney failure is still tough. Dialysis is now available to anyone who needs and wants it - and the opportunities for having dialysis at home are now better than ever. More living donor kidney transplantation is being done, and new technologies are emerging that enable more people to benefit from a transplant.

We hope that, armed with information, patients and their loved ones, can get the best health for themselves, and work to improve things for others.

Andy Stein and Janet Wild

DEDICATION

This book is dedicated to the tens of thousands
of patients with kidney failure in the UK.
Their will to live has inspired us all.

1 WHAT IS KIDNEY FAILURE?

This first chapter begins by explaining how kidneys work. Then it explores what goes wrong when someone has chronic kidney failure, what causes this problem and why it should be treated.

INTRODUCTION

Chronic kidney failure is a serious, long-term medical condition. At the present time, there are approximately 45,500 people in the UK who are either on dialysis or have received a kidney transplant to treat chronic kidney failure. Of these, 43% are on haemodialysis, 10% on peritoneal dialysis (PD) and 47% have a transplant. This is just over one person in 1,350, making it a rare condition. This means that a typical family doctor will have only one or two kidney patients 'on their books'.

Chronic kidney failure has many possible causes, but the effects are usually the same. The kidneys become less and less able to do their normal work. After a time, the kidneys stop working almost completely – a condition known as end-stage renal failure (ESRF), end-stage renal disease (ESRD) or end-stage kidney failure. You may hear any one of these names for kidney failure, but the most widely used term now is established renal failure, or ERF.

There are approximately 6,500 new patients diagnosed with ERF every year.

When the kidneys stop working in this way, treatment that takes over the work they do becomes essential. The main treatments are dialysis – either peritoneal dialysis (PD) or haemodialysis which can be done either at home or in the renal unit – and transplantation. These treatments cannot 'cure' kidney failure, but they can improve health and prolong life.

KIDNEYS – WHAT AND WHERE ARE THEY?

Most people have two kidneys. These important body organs are shaped like beans and are about 12 centimetres (5 inches) long, which is about the length of a man's palm. They are approximately 6 centimetres wide and 3 centimetres thick. Each kidney weighs about 150 grams (6 ounces). The kidneys sit under the lower ribs at the back, one on either side of the body (see *diagram* on next page).

The kidneys lie deep inside the body, so you cannot normally 'feel' them.

THE KIDNEYS' MAIN JOB: MAKING URINE

The main job of the kidneys is to be the body's dustmen. They clean up the blood and make urine from the waste products they take out of it. When urine is passed, the rubbish is taken away. How does this happen?

Blood is pumped by the heart to the kidneys. Each kidney has a drainage system that takes urine from that kidney to the bladder. This drainage system is like a funnel with a tube (the ureter) that connects the kidney to the bladder (see *diagram* on next page). Urine passes down the ureters (one for each kidney) into the bladder.

Urine is stored in the bladder before being passed from the body via another tube, called the urethra. The

Location of kidneys and urinary system

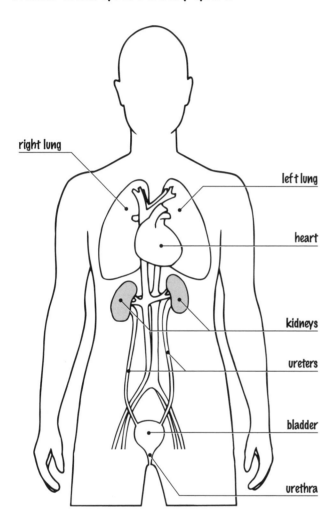

- right lung
- left lung
- heart
- kidneys
- ureters
- bladder
- urethra

bladder holds about 400 ml (¾ pint) of urine when 'full'.

But when you have just emptied it, by going to the toilet, it will be almost completely empty.

People normally pass around 2 litres (4 pints) of urine per day.

WHY MAKE URINE?

The kidneys make urine in order to perform their two most important functions. These are:

1. Removing wastes from the blood – a process called 'clearance'. (See *below* for a brief description, and *Chapter 2* for more details.)

2. Removing excess salt and water from the body – a process called 'ultrafiltration'. (See *page 3* for a brief description, and *Chapter 3* for more details.)

REMOVING WASTES

The kidneys play a very important role in getting rid of waste products. The food we eat is normally digested in the stomach and the bowels. During digestion, the food is broken down into substances that can be carried around the body in the blood. These 'good things' in the bloodstream provide every part of the body with the energy it needs to work, and with the substances necessary for growth and repair.

When the different parts of the body make use of the various 'good things' in the blood, they also produce waste products. These wastes are toxic (poisonous) to the body and make people unwell unless they are removed. Like the 'good things', these 'bad things' also travel around the body in the bloodstream.

When the waste products of food in the blood reach the kidneys, it is the job of the kidneys to get rid of them in the urine. What the kidneys do is to sieve and filter the blood, removing the wastes and putting them in the urine, but leaving the 'good things' in the blood. Healthy kidneys generally have no problems getting rid of all the many waste products normally produced by the body.

In people with kidney failure, however, the levels of waste products build up in the blood. It is this build-up of waste products that makes people with kidney failure feel unwell. When someone is in the early stages of

A kidney

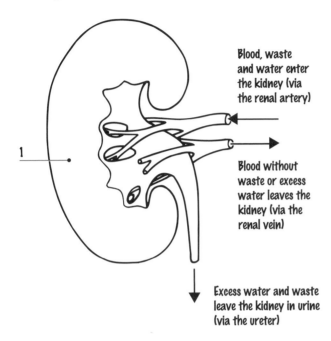

Blood, waste and water enter the kidney (via the renal artery)

Blood without waste or excess water leaves the kidney (via the renal vein)

Excess water and waste leave the kidney in urine (via the ureter)

1 In this part of the kidney there are 1,000,000 filtering units (nephrons)

kidney failure, there are usually no symptoms, because the levels of waste products are not high enough to cause them. (This can be true even when the kidneys are working at less than 25% of their normal capacity.)

REMOVING EXCESS WATER

The second most important function of the kidneys is to remove excess water from the body. As well as getting rid of the waste products of food, healthy kidneys also remove excess fluids from the body. Like the food that we eat, the water (and tea, coffee, beer and all other liquids) that we drink is digested into the stomach and bowels and absorbed into the blood. When the blood reaches the

kidneys, the normal sieving and filtering process removes any excess water and puts it in the urine. So normal urine contains not only the waste products of food, but also any excess water that has been drunk.

When kidneys fail, they are unable to remove excess water from the bloodstream. People with established

A kidney filtering unit (nephron)

1 Blood from the renal artery (a) is filtered inside a glomerulus (b)

2 Water and waste products filtered from the blood enter a tube system (c)

3 Blood vessels (d) take most of the water back around the body via the renal vein (e)

4 Waste products and excess water (the urine) are removed via a drainage duct (f) that eventually drains into the bladder

kidney failure don't usually pass much urine. Excess fluid can therefore build up in the body, causing it to become 'waterlogged' – a condition called fluid overload (see *Chapter 3*). This will eventually lead to swelling of the ankles, and shortness of breath due to excess fluid in the lungs.

OTHER FUNCTIONS OF THE KIDNEYS

As well as water and waste removal, the kidneys have three important 'extra' functions. These are:

1. Helping to control blood pressure. The blood pressure is finely controlled by healthy kidneys. When someone's kidneys fail, their blood pressure usually goes up. High blood pressure is unlikely to cause symptoms unless the pressure gets very high, but it increases the risk of a stroke or heart attack, and can cause the kidneys to deteriorate more rapidly (see also *Chapter 4*).

2. Helping to control the manufacture of red blood cells. The kidneys help control the making of red blood cells in the bone marrow (the runny bit in the middle of all bones). The red blood cells float in the liquid part of the blood (called plasma). Their job is to carry oxygen around the body. Every part of the body needs oxygen to function properly.

When someone has kidney failure, they make fewer red blood cells than normal. This causes them to become anaemic (i.e. they are short of red blood cells). This anaemia contributes to the tiredness suffered by most people with kidney failure – it is not only high waste levels that cause tiredness. (See *Chapter 5* for more about anaemia and how it can be treated.)

3. Helping to keep the bones strong and healthy. Calcium and phosphate are two minerals found in the blood and in the bones. If the bones are to stay strong and healthy, there must be a correct balance between these minerals in the body. The kidneys help to maintain this balance. When someone develops kidney failure, the normal balance between calcium and phosphate in the body is lost. The level of calcium in the blood goes down, while the level of phosphate in the blood goes up. Unless this imbalance is treated, it will result in a condition called renal bone disease. This may cause aches and pains in the bones, and even fractures. (See *Chapter 6* for more information about renal bone disease and its treatment.)

KIDNEY FAILURE – WHAT IS IT?

In short, kidney failure is a condition in which the kidneys are less able than normal to perform their usual functions. These functions are:

- removing waste products from the body;
- removing excess water;
- helping to control blood pressure;
- helping to control red blood cell manufacture; and
- helping to keep the bones strong and healthy.

This book is about the long-term condition known as chronic kidney failure or chronic renal failure. There is a more modern phrase, chronic kidney disease (CKD). Currently, it is thought that chronic kidney 'disease' becomes chronic kidney 'failure' when the kidney function is less than 60%. There is a separate condition, known as acute kidney failure, in which the kidneys suddenly stop working. Short-term treatment may be needed for acute kidney failure, but the kidneys usually get better on their own. This book does not tell you about acute kidney failure.

When someone's kidneys start to fail, their kidneys become less and less able to do their work. This happens gradually, usually over a period of many years. Eventually, the kidneys stop working almost completely

– a condition called established renal failure or ERF. Treatment is then essential to take over the work of the kidneys and so keep the patient alive. The treatments for ERF are dialysis or a kidney transplant (see *page 1*).

WHAT ARE THE SYMPTOMS?

In the early stages of chronic kidney failure, there are often no symptoms. Later, the condition may cause any of the following:

- itching;
- weakness or tiredness;
- loss of appetite;
- poor concentration;
- restless legs;
- leg cramps;
- swollen ankles;
- shortness of breath;
- poor sleeping;
- low sex drive; and
- feeling cold.

HOW IS KIDNEY FAILURE DIAGNOSED?

Kidney failure is diagnosed by measuring kidney function. A reliable way to measure kidney function is to measure the levels of a substance called creatinine in a patient's blood. Creatinine is one of the many waste products that build up in the blood when someone has kidney disease. Creatinine is produced when muscles are used and can be measured from a blood sample. The higher the creatinine level, the worse the kidney function. The normal level of creatinine is between 50 and 120 µmol/l (micromoles per litre of blood), depending on your weight, gender and size.

Many renal units then calculate an estimate of kidney function using the creatinine and the patient's gender, weight, age and ethnic origin. This is known as an estimated glomerular filtration rate, or eGFR. The eGFR is roughly equivalent to the percentage function the kidney has compared to a healthy kidney.

- **If a person's creatinine is over 150 µmol/l, or their eGFR goes below 60 mls/min (i.e. 60%), they have kidney failure** (see *Chapter 2*).

As soon as your creatinine level starts to rise, and your eGFR to go below 60, your GP should monitor your health and your kidney function on a regular basis to make sure that serious disease is not beginning to develop.

Creatinine testing is used not only to detect kidney failure, but also used at all stages of kidney disease – before dialysis, during dialysis and after a transplant. The amount of creatinine in the blood is the single most important piece of information that doctors and nurses require when looking after people with kidney failure. (See *Chapter 2* for more information.)

If you have kidney failure, you should know what your blood creatinine level is all the time. Ask the nurse to tell you the value each time you have a blood test.

WHAT CAUSES KIDNEYS TO FAIL?

There are hundreds of different diseases that can cause kidneys to start failing, and sometimes to fail completely. Usually, however, ERF (leading to dialysis or a transplant) is likely to be due to one of the following causes:

1. Diabetes mellitus. Diabetes is the most common known cause of kidney failure in the developed world where it may be the cause of ERF in up to 40% of patients in some countries.

Whether diabetes is controlled by insulin, tablets or diet, it can cause kidney failure (known as diabetic nephropathy). This is more likely to happen when someone has had diabetes for more than 10 years. In the UK, an average of 22% of new dialysis patients *every* year are thought to be suffering from diabetic nephropathy.

The only way of definitely diagnosing this condition is by kidney biopsy (see *page 46*). But this procedure carries some risk, so it is not done routinely for *every* patient.

2. Nephritis. The term 'nephritis' means inflammation of the kidneys ('neph' means 'kidney', and 'it is' means 'inflammation'). The term is usually applied to people with glomerulonephritis or GN. ('Glomerulo' refers to the glomeruli, which are part of the kidneys' filtration unit.)

The causes of most types of nephritis are unknown. Nephritis is another condition that can only be diagnosed for certain by a kidney biopsy (see *page 46*).

3. Polycystic kidney disease (PCKD). This is an inherited disease (a disease that runs in families) in which both kidneys become filled ('poly' means 'many') with cysts (abnormal fluid-filled lumps). If someone has PCKD, they will have a 50% chance of passing the condition on to each of their children.

PCKD is diagnosed by ultrasound (an investigation that uses sound waves to produce a picture of the kidneys). Polycystic kidneys, although abnormally large because of the cysts, do not work well. Many people with PCKD eventually develop ERF.

The cysts in PCKD can remain a problem after treatment for kidney failure has started. A cyst can burst, bleed or get infected – any of which may cause pain. Occasionally, a large cyst that is particularly troublesome will have to be drained through a long, hollow needle inserted into the patient, or removed by an operation.

Sometimes, people with polycystic kidneys have to have one of them removed to make room for a transplanted kidney.

4. Pyelonephritis. 'Pyelo' (meaning 'funnel') refers to the drainage system of the kidney and 'nephritis' means 'kidney inflammation', so pyelonephritis means 'inflammation of the kidney drainage system'. Pyelonephritis is diagnosed by ultrasound, or by a special X-ray of the kidneys called an intravenous pyelogram (IVP), in which an opaque dye is injected into the bloodstream. It can also be diagnosed by a special nuclear medicine scan of the kidneys (called a DMSA or MAG-3 scan), in which a small amount of a radioactive substance is injected into the bloodstream.

Pyelonephritis can sometimes be linked to repeated kidney infections. These may have gone undetected for many years, perhaps having occurred in childhood.

Pyelonephritis is sometimes caused by a condition called reflux nephropathy (or 'reflux'). In this condition, a valve where the ureter enters the bladder (see *diagram, page 2*) is faulty. This faulty valve allows urine from the bladder to flow back up the ureter to cause problems in the kidney.

Reflux is a partially inherited condition, particularly in women. So the children of patients with reflux should be tested for it soon after birth. This is true for boys and girls, whichever parent has the condition.

5. Renovascular disease. As people get older, their arteries tend to become 'furred' up with cholesterol and other fats. Diabetes and smoking make this process occur at a younger age. This 'furring up' (which is called atheroma or atherosclerosis) gradually narrows the arteries (the blood vessels that take blood from the heart to every part of the body).

Atheroma in the arteries that supply the heart's own muscle leads to angina and heart attacks. If the atheroma affects the arteries that supply blood to the brain, it may cause a stroke. Atheroma can also affect and block the arteries that supply blood to the kidneys, the renal arteries. This is called renovascular disease ('reno' means kidney, and 'vascular' means blood vessel). Renovascular disease is a particularly common cause of kidney failure in older patients. A renal angiogram (see *page 48*) is the only way of definitely diagnosing the condition. But this procedure carries some risk, so it is not done routinely for every patient.

6. Obstructive nephropathy. This is a common cause of ERF in men, especially those over the age of 60 years. It is usually due to enlargement of the prostate gland, which obstructs the urethra (hence the name 'obstructive nephropathy'). The urethra is the tube through which the urine drains from the bladder.

Surgery to the prostate gland (even if it is enlarged due to cancer) can often reverse the kidney failure. But in some people, especially those who were diagnosed late, ERF requiring dialysis or a transplant will occur, even if the patient has had an operation on the prostate to relieve the blockage.

7. Unknown. In about 25% of patients with ERF, the cause of the kidney failure is never discovered. This is because the kidneys often appear small and shrunken when shown by ultrasound. For this reason, a diagnosis of 'two small kidneys' is often made. 'Two small kidneys' really means that the kidneys are small, but doctors don't know why. It is presumed that 'something' happened to the kidneys years ago, and they have slowly shrivelled up since.

THE 'PROGRESSION' OF KIDNEY FAILURE

When chronic kidney failure is still at an early stage, most patients feel quite well. This is because their failing kidneys 'overwork' to keep the level of body waste normal. This hides the fact that the kidneys are failing.

In other words, the kidneys have a lot 'in reserve'. The body manages for quite some time to adapt to high levels of waste products and excess water in the blood. It does this by making the kidneys work harder.

The rate at which kidney disease gets worse varies from patient to patient. Also, the symptoms that patients get when they have similar levels of kidney function can vary considerably. Some patients get symptoms when their kidney function is 75% of normal, whereas others do not get symptoms until their kidney function is down to 5% of normal!

However, for most people, the stages of their kidney disease will be as shown in the table overleaf. Stages 1, 2 and 3 do not necessarily progress to ERF. However, if you are reading this book it is likely that you or someone you care about has Stage 4 kidney disease or worse.

If someone has Stage 4 kidney disease – whatever its cause – it is likely that their kidneys will eventually stop working completely. Doctors do not know why failing kidneys usually get worse, or why people with chronic kidney failure usually progress to ERF.

WHAT IS ERF?

This is surprisingly difficult to define. However, most doctors would say that ERF has occurred when treatment by dialysis or a transplant becomes essential for life. When kidney failure is 'established', it very rarely gets better. Once someone develops ERF, they will always have it, even after they have had a transplant (see *Chapter 11*).

If the kidneys start to fail in an older person (say, in someone over 70 years old), that person may live out their natural lifespan without experiencing any problems from their kidneys. This is because the kidneys can take up to 10 years to progress to ERF. So, sometimes, older people never need treatment for their kidney failure. If an older person develops ERF, however, they can still be treated by dialysis or a transplant.

THE STAGES AND SIGNS OF KIDNEY DISEASE

CKD Stage	Creatinine	eGFR	Dialysis?	Description	Symptoms	Treatment	Progression
1	<120	90–99	No	Near-normal kidney function but urine findings or structural abnormalities or genetic traits point to kidney disease	Well	Observation, control of blood pressure and risk factors	Usually does not progress or worsen
2	120–150	60–89	Rarely	Mildly reduced kidney function, and other findings (as for Stage 1) point to kidney disease	Well	Observation, control of blood pressure and risk factors	May not progress
3	150–250	30–59	In 1–5 years, or never	Moderately reduced kidney function	Symptoms variable	Consider need for established renal failure treatment	May progress
4	250–400	15–29	In 6–24 months	Severely reduced kidney function	Often unwell	Planning established renal failure treatment	Usually progresses
5	>400	<15	In less than 6 months	Very severe established or end stage renal failure	Unwell	Make treatment choice	Progresses
	>500	<5	Immediate	Life in danger	Severe and unpleasant	Treatment essential	

The Stages 1–5 which form part of this table are based on the KDOQI CKD Guidelines developed in the USA in 2002.

HOW IS ERF TREATED?

ERF can be treated by dialysis or by a kidney transplant. It is usual for a patient to undergo a period of dialysis before transplantation is considered. Dialysis and transplantation provide alternative ways of taking over the work of the patient's failed kidneys:

1. Dialysis. In this treatment, some of the work of the kidneys is performed by artificial means. (See *Chapter 8* for a description of what dialysis is and how it works.) There are two main types of dialysis: PD and haemo-dialysis. (PD is described in detail in *Chapter 9,* and haemodialysis in *Chapter 10.*) Either PD or haemo-dialysis usually provides about 5% of the function of two normal kidneys.

2. Transplantation. This treatment involves the removal of a healthy kidney from one person (the donor), and its insertion into a patient with kidney failure (the recipient). Transplantation is done by a surgeon during a transplant operation. A 'good' transplant provides 50–60% of the function of two healthy kidneys. (Transplantation is described in *Chapter 11.*)

WHEN SHOULD DIALYSIS BE STARTED?

Dialysis is usually started either when:

- a patient has symptoms of kidney failure which affect normal daily life; or
- the levels of waste products and/or excess water in the body are so high that they become life-threatening.

An eGFR of 15 mls/minute or less is generally taken to indicate Stage 5 kidney failure, and the time at which the need for dialysis is becoming imminent. However, the actual level at which dialysis is started varies from patient to patient (*see Chapter 2*). Most doctors now usually try to start patients on dialysis when their eGFR is 5–10 mls/minute, depending on their symptoms. Individual decisions always take into account the patient's condition, and their wishes, not just the eGFR alone.

CAN THE NEED FOR DIALYSIS BE DELAYED?

Once a patient has developed ERF, dialysis should be started very soon. However, if someone with chronic kidney disease has not yet developed ERF, it may sometimes be possible to delay the need for dialysis.

This is particularly true for Stages 1, 2 and 3 of kidney disease, which can often be held 'in check' for years so the patient never progresses to Stage 4 or beyond.

The following treatments may delay the need for dialysis or a transplant in some patients:

1. Treatments to control blood pressure. High blood pressure is known to speed up kidney failure. Doctors therefore make great efforts to keep the blood pressure of their kidney patients low. Keeping the blood pressure low (consistently 130/80 mmHg or less) can delay the need for dialysis by years. This is true for most patients with kidney failure – the cause of the kidney failure makes no difference. (See *Chapter 4* for more about blood pressure and kidney failure.)

2. Treatments to slow down the underlying kidney disease. When kidney failure is due to nephritis (*see page 6*), the need for dialysis can sometimes be delayed by tablets called immuno-suppressants. In some types of nephritis, the body's immune system (the system that normally fights infection or foreign objects in the body) starts to attack the patient's kidneys and stops them working properly. So tablets that make the immune system less effective – such as the steroid tablet called prednisolone – can be used to treat the kidney problem. In some patients, such treatments are very successful, and return the kidney function to normal or near normal. In other patients, these tablets are less successful. Even so, they may delay the need for dialysis or a transplant by many years. (There is more information on the immune system in *Chapter 13*.)

3. Use of ACE inhibitors/A2-antagonists. This is a more controversial treatment that may delay the need for dialysis or a transplant in some patients. Some people with kidney failure (especially kidney failure caused by diabetes or nephritis) have a large amount of protein in the urine. Normally, there is next-to-no protein in the urine. If a kidney patient has a raised level of protein in the urine, doctors often attempt to reduce it with a type of blood pressure tablet called an ACE inhibitor or ARB. Whether this treatment in fact delays the need to start dialysis is not yet proven.

4. Treating obstructive nephropathy. This is the only cause of ERF that can, in many cases, be wholly or partially reversed. Initially, this is done either by putting a plastic tube (urinary catheter) into the bladder through the urethra; or one or more tubes (nephrostomies) through the skin, into the pelvis (drainage system) of the kidney. Depending on the cause of the obstruction, these procedures in men are usually followed by an operation on the prostate gland, after which the plastic tubes can usually be taken out.

Women do not have a prostate gland, so obstruction in a woman would be caused by something else.

WILL DIALYSIS OR A TRANSPLANT SOLVE THE PROBLEM?

Neither dialysis nor a kidney transplant can 'cure' a patient with ERF. These treatments can control the symptoms of kidney failure, but they cannot get rid of the symptoms completely nor restore the kidneys to health.

1. Dialysis. When someone is treated by dialysis, the symptoms of kidney failure never really go away completely. This is because either type of dialysis – PD (see *Chapter 9*) or haemodialysis (see *Chapter 10*) – can provide only about 5% of the function of two normal kidneys. So when a patient starts dialysis, they will usually have only about 10% of the function of two normal kidneys (5% from dialysis, and 5% from their own kidneys). This is simply not enough to make the person feel completely better. Hence on dialysis the creatinine level usually settles to 500–600 µmol/l before dialysis on haemodialysis, and all the time for patients on PD.

The symptoms of kidney failure will also tend to worsen if the person is not getting enough dialysis. It is important that sufficient dialysis is given to bring the amount of creatinine in a patient's blood down to target level (see *Chapter 2* for more information).

Even though dialysis technology has its limitations, it does do a reasonable job. So it is sensible to start treatment as early as possible – before a patient becomes very unwell. This means that some patients may feel relatively well when they start dialysis. The doctor will be able to tell from a patient's blood creatinine, eGFR and symptoms when is the best time to start dialysis.

2. Transplantation. A kidney transplant is more effective than dialysis at removing the symptoms of kidney failure. This is because a transplanted kidney can provide up to 60% of the function of two normal kidneys. It can be 60% rather than 50% as the new kidney has the potential to grow and overwork. So the patient settles back into Stage 2 or 3 kidney disease with a creatinine of 120–250µmol/l. A stable creatinine of this level indicates a 'good' transplant.

However, transplants often have their own problems. They do not last for ever and it may be necessary for a patient to have a second transplant or to resume dialysis if the transplant fails. (*See Chapters 11–13* for more information about transplantation.)

WHY TREAT KIDNEY FAILURE?

If someone with ERF is not treated by dialysis or a transplant, they will develop *severe kidney failure symptoms* (see *page 5*), and then, after a few weeks, they will die.

Given the terrible result if no treatment is given, it may seem stupid to ask: 'Why treat kidney failure?' The answer seems obvious – 'to keep patients alive'. To a certain extent this is true. When people have ERF, they will die without treatment.

So, certainly, the main purpose of the treatment of ERF is to keep patients alive. However, there is little point in keeping patients alive if their quality of life is so poor that they don't want to be alive.

There are, in fact, several reasons why treatment is given to patients with kidney failure. Firstly, treatment prolongs life in most people. Secondly, it aims to make patients feel better, and to return them to a good quality of life. To achieve this, the two main functions of the kidneys – removing toxins (see *Chapter 2*) and maintaining the body's fluid balance (see *Chapter 3*) – have to be performed for the patient. Dialysis and transplantation can perform both these vital functions.

Some very elderly and frail patients occasionally decide that dialysis is too much of a burden for them. They, and the people who care for them, may feel that the extra months or years of life that dialysis offers may not compensate for the responsibility and inconvenience it causes. In these patients, medicines such as ESAs are given to help control symptoms until the patient eventually dies.

KEY FACTS

1 The two main functions of your kidneys are:
   - removing waste products;
   - removing excess water and salt.

2 If your kidneys are failing, they will be less able to carry out these functions.

3 Whatever the original cause of your kidney failure, it is likely to get worse over a period of years.

4 A special test (the eGFR) is used to measure the amount of work that the kidneys can still do. This is normally about 100 mls/min, equivalent to 100% of kidney function. If it is less than 60 mls/min (i.e. 60%) you have kidney failure.

5 Many people with chronic (Stage 4) kidney disease (eGFR <30 mls/min, i.e. <30%) will go on to develop ERF, when they will need dialysis or a transplant.

6 For most kidney patients, good control of blood pressure is essential to delay the onset of ERF and the need for dialysis.

7 The treatment of kidney failure (by dialysis or transplantation) is effective, but it is not a 'cure' and may not get rid of all the symptoms.

2 CLEARANCE

This chapter looks at ways of measuring the ability of the kidneys, or dialysis, to remove (or 'clear') waste products from the blood.

INTRODUCTION

One of the main functions of the kidneys is to remove the waste products of food from the blood. This function is sometimes called 'clearance', because waste is 'cleared' away. When someone has kidney failure, their kidneys become less efficient at clearing waste products from the blood. This leads to a build-up of harmful waste products in the blood. It is this build-up that makes people with kidney failure feel unwell. Doctors do not know which particular waste products make people ill.

WHY IS CLEARANCE MEASURED?

Tests that indicate the clearance of waste from the blood are extremely important when someone has kidney failure.

Clearance measurements are used:

- in the diagnosis of kidney failure;
- to find out how severe the kidney failure is;
- to decide whether it is time for a patient to start treatment by dialysis;
- to monitor treatment by dialysis; and
- to assess how well a transplant is working.

Clearance provides a more reliable guide to a kidney patient's condition than is possible from either a physical examination or an account of the patient's symptoms. Some patients get a lot of symptoms when their kidney function is not too bad. Others get few or no symptoms even when doctors and nurses think that they need dialysis.

HOW IS CLEARANCE MEASURED?

There are tens of thousands of different substances in the blood. Fortunately, there is no need to measure most of them. The overall ability of the kidneys to clear wastes from the blood is assessed by measuring the blood levels of two particular substances. These are called urea and creatinine:

1. Urea is a waste product produced by the liver. When we eat protein (such as in meat and eggs), the body uses this protein (in the form of amino acids) to repair itself and to build muscles. The 'used' proteins are then taken in the blood to the liver, where they are changed into urea. The urea then travels in the blood to the kidneys, where it enters the urine.

2. Creatinine is a substance created by the muscles whenever they are used. The harder our muscles work, the more creatinine they produce. This is a little bit like a car engine producing exhaust fumes. So our muscles are like the engine which drives the car, and creatinine is like the exhaust from the engine. Like urea, creatinine is carried in the blood to the kidneys, where it is filtered and enters the urine.

Creatinine production

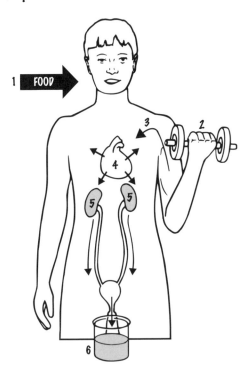

1 Protein is eaten in food
2 Protein is used to make strong muscles
3 Creatinine is produced in the muscles when they are used
4 Creatinine is pumped around the body in the bloodstream by the heart
5 Blood is filtered in the kidneys
6 Creatinine is passed in urine along with other waste products

WHY MEASURE UREA OR CREATININE?

Normal healthy kidneys can remove both urea and creatinine from the body quite well. However, when someone has kidney failure, the blood levels of both these substances rise above normal:

- **The normal blood level of urea** is between 2.6 and 6.6 mmol/l (millimoles of urea per litre of blood).

- **The normal blood level of creatinine** is between 50 and 120 µmol/l (micromoles of creatinine per litre of blood).

Urea and creatinine are not, in themselves, particularly harmful to the body. Creatinine is not even a toxin. However, tests that indicate the clearance of urea and creatinine from the body provide an indication of the clearance of all the thousands of other harmful substances that are produced by the body. In kidney failure, there is a build-up of urea, creatinine and all these waste products.

A substance which is known to indicate the presence of another substance or condition is called a 'marker'. Urea and creatinine do not themselves make people with kidney failure feel ill. However, both urea and creatinine are markers for the many more harmful waste products that do make kidney patients feel ill.

TYPES OF TEST

Different tests show how well or badly the kidneys (or dialysis or a transplanted kidney) are managing to clear the blood of urea or creatinine.

There are basically three types of test:

- **blood tests,** which measure the level of urea or creatinine in the blood (see *page 14*);

- **clearance tests,** which measure the amount of urea or creatinine removed from the blood (see *pages 16–17*);

- **the eGFR,** which measures how many millilitres of blood the kidney is able to filter (and thus 'clean up') in a minute. This gives a good indication of how efficiently the kidneys are working.

BLOOD TESTS FOR UREA OR CREATININE

Blood tests provide a direct measurement of the levels of urea or creatinine present in a patient's blood. These levels can then be compared with normal levels (see *page 13*), or with a range of expected or target levels at different stages of a patient's illness or treatment (see *page 8*).

In simple terms, the higher the levels of urea or creatinine in a patient's blood, the worse the kidney (dialysis or transplant) function. The lower the levels, the better.

In reality, the picture is not quite so simple. Blood urea tests are not always a reliable guide to a patient's kidney function. This is because blood urea levels are affected by things other than the kidneys, such as the amount of protein in the diet. Blood creatinine tests are a generally more reliable guide to kidney function, and have now largely replaced blood urea tests.

It is also the case that blood levels of both urea and creatinine are affected by an individual's overall size and muscle bulk. Larger and more muscular people have higher blood levels of creatinine and urea than smaller and less muscular people. This is true both when someone is healthy and at all stages of kidney failure. Overall size and muscle bulk must therefore be taken into account when looking at an individual's blood urea and blood creatinine test results.

BLOOD CREATININE BEFORE DIALYSIS

Blood tests that measure the level of creatinine in a patient's blood provide doctors with the information they need to decide:

- whether a patient has kidney failure; and

- how bad it is.

The normal level of creatinine in the blood is known to be between 50 and 120 µmol/l. So, if anyone has a creatinine level of over 120 µmol/l, it means that they have reduced kidney function.

As stated above, the normal level for any particular individual depends on their overall size and muscle bulk. For example, a healthy large man might have a normal blood creatinine of 120 µmol/l (at the top of the normal range). However, the same blood creatinine of 120 µmol/l in a small woman might indicate the start of kidney failure; her normal blood creatinine might be as low as 40 µmol/l (below the bottom level of the normal range).

At the start of kidney failure, the blood creatinine level tends to increase slowly over time. This can take months, or, more often, many years. However, when the kidneys have almost completely failed, the blood creatinine level rises more rapidly. Patients will probably start to feel unwell when their creatinine level gets to more than about 250 µmol/l, equivalent to about 30% of normal kidney function (i.e. chronic kidney disease Stage 4). At a creatinine level of 400 µmol/l (i.e. less than 15% function or chronic kidney failure Stage 5) almost all patients will feel very unwell.

It is not quite as simple as this, unfortunately. As, at all stages of kidney failure, large patients will have a relatively higher blood creatinine than small patients. So, for example, a large man whose kidney function is only 25% of normal could have a creatinine level of 400 µmol/l. But a small woman who has 25% of normal kidney function could have a creatinine level of 250 µmol/l.

STARTING DIALYSIS

Dialysis is usually started when a patient's blood creatinine is more than 500 µmol/l. At this stage, the eGFR is likely to be <5 mls/minute (i.e. less than 5% function). Unless someone with kidney failure starts dialysis at this point, they will become very unwell.

The actual creatinine level or eGFR at which any patient starts dialysis will take into account their size and muscle bulk, as well as the degree to which they are troubled by symptoms of kidney failure and feeling generally unwell. Guidelines are based on the needs of an 'average' person, but most people are not average. So the precise levels for starting dialysis are different for different patients.

BLOOD CREATININE DURING DIALYSIS

Measurement of blood creatinine continues to be important after a patient has started dialysis. This applies to patients on either type of dialysis – peritoneal dialysis (PD) (see *Chapter 9*) or haemodialysis (see *Chapter* 10).

Blood creatinine level provides vital information about how well dialysis is working. A 'high' level of creatinine could mean that a patient is not getting enough dialysis – i.e. dialysis is not removing enough waste products.

When planning an individual patient's treatment, doctors and nurses aim to keep the patient's blood creatinine at or below recognised 'target' levels. These targets take into account both the size of the patient and the type of dialysis.

The following table summarises the target creatinine levels for different sizes of patient:

Weight	Target creatinine
Less than 60 kg	Less than 500 μmol/l
60–90 kg	Less than 600 μmol/l
More than 90 kg	Less than 800 μmol/l

A blood creatinine of 600 μmol/l is the accepted target level for a person of average size and muscle bulk.

The fact that the creatinine target levels are the same for PD and haemodialysis indicates that the two techniques provide roughly the same amount of dialysis. One is not 'better' than the other.

The creatinine level in a PD patient will almost remain constant, because PD is a continuous treatment. However, haemodialysis is done intermittently, usually just three times a week, and so the level of creatinine goes up and down between each dialysis session. Haemodialysis will remove a lot of creatinine, so the level in the blood straight after a dialysis session will be lower that it was at the start. For this reason, the 'target' creatinine of 600 μmol/l is for blood that is sampled before the start of dialysis.

If dialysis does not achieve creatinine target levels over a period of time, the patient will be in danger of, once again, developing the symptoms of kidney failure. This problem is called under-dialysis.

Under-dialysis is corrected by increasing the amount of dialysis. Ways of doing this are described in later chapters (see *Chapter 9* for PD, and *Chapter 10* for haemodialysis).

BLOOD CREATININE WITH A TRANSPLANT

Ideally, the blood creatinine of an average-sized person with a transplanted kidney should be less than 120 μmol/l (i.e. the upper limit of normal). However, even if a transplant is working well, the blood creatinine may not return to a normal level. This is because the maximum function it can provide is 50–60% of normal.

So the creatinine usually settles to around 120–250 μmol/l (i.e. Stages 2–3 kidney disease). A creatinine level of below 150 μmol/l is generally considered satisfactory for a patient in this situation, so long as it is stable.

If a transplanted kidney starts to fail, the patient's blood creatinine level will rise again. When it exceeds

500 µmol/l (<5% function), it is probably time to start dialysis again. The creatinine level for restarting dialysis is therefore the same as the level at which a patient who is new to kidney failure would start on dialysis. This is because the period in which a transplant fails is very similar to the period before dialysis is first started.

UREA OR CREATININE CLEARANCE TESTS

Most renal units now use tests called urea or creatinine clearance tests in addition to blood tests for measuring their patients' kidney (dialysis or transplant) function.

Urea or creatinine clearance tests are sometimes preferred to simple blood tests because they link the amount of urea or creatinine in a patient's blood to the size of the patient's body and muscles. In some situations, this may make these tests a more reliable measure of the effectiveness of dialysis.

The test used to measure the clearance of urea is called urea kinetic modelling. The amount of urea clearance is expressed in terms of Kt/V (pronounced 'K…t…over V').

The clearance of creatinine is measured in millilitres per minute (ml/min) or litres per day (l/d) or week (l/wk).

Blood tests measure the levels of waste products remaining in the blood. So, when blood urea or blood creatinine is measured, the lower the number the better. High numbers reflect poor kidney (dialysis or transplant) function.

The opposite is true for eGFR than for urea and creatinine clearance measurements. Low numbers reflect poor kidney function. This is because clearance (or eGFR) tests measure the amount of toxin *removed* from the blood. So, for clearance test results, the higher the number, the better. A low number indicates poor functioning of the kidneys (or dialysis or transplant).

When the blood creatinine is down to 500 µmol/l (after the onset of ERF), the creatinine clearance is usually down to about 5 ml/min (i.e. about 5% of normal).

Dialysis provides about 5 ml/min of creatinine clearance (i.e. about 5% of normal). So, when a patient starts dialysis, the combined effort of the kidneys and dialysis is only about 10% of what two normal kidneys can do. This is why patients with kidney failure rarely feel perfectly well on dialysis. Neither PD nor haemodialysis is good enough at clearing wastes.

HOW IS CLEARANCE MEASURED?

Different methods for measuring the clearance of urea or creatinine are used for different patients, depending on their type of treatment:

1. Patients not on dialysis. Clearance of urea or creatinine in these patients (either pre-dialysis or with a transplant) is measured by comparing:

- the amount of urea or creatinine passed in the patient's urine over a period of 24 hours; with

- the amount of urea or creatinine in the patient's blood.

To provide accurate results, it is essential that the collection of urine is done very carefully. Every drop of urine collected in the 24-hour period must be collected, otherwise the information will be less reliable than that gained from simple blood urea or blood creatinine tests. Because of this, many doctors now prefer an estimated glomerular filtration rate test or eGFR (see below) that does not need a urine collection.

2. PD patients. In PD patients, clearance is measured by measuring:

- the amount of urea or creatinine in 24 hours' worth of the patient's used dialysis fluid,

- plus the amount of urea or creatinine in 24 hours' worth of urine that they might pass;

and comparing that with

- the patient's blood urea or creatinine level (taking into account the patient's size).

3. Haemodialysis patients.
For haemodialysis patients, the most accurate method is to calculate the urea reduction ratio (URR) by comparing:

- the patient's blood urea level before dialysis; with

- the patient's blood urea level after dialysis.

When measuring clearance in dialysis patients, it is also necessary to take into account patient size, as well as the urea or creatinine passed in the urine.

People who have PD are more likely to maintain some kidney function for up to two years after the start of dialysis, meaning that they will continue to pass urine. Haemodialysis, when it's done intermittently, three times a week, can cause the complete loss of any kidney function. This means that many people having haemodialysis will stop passing any urine within a few months of starting treatment.

Urea or creatinine clearance during dialysis
When monitoring urea or creatinine clearance in a dialysis patient, doctors and nurses will compare that patient's levels with generally accepted levels for patients on dialysis. The current guidelines state that:

PD patients should have:

- a creatinine clearance of 50 l/wk (litres per week); and

- a urea clearance (Kt/V) of 1.7 l/wk.

Haemodialysis patients should have:

- a urea reduction ratio (URR) of greater than 65%; and

- a urea clearance (Kt/V) of 1.2 for each dialysis session.

These goals are the same for all patients as they take into account size and build, as well as the amount of waste that patients can get rid of through their own kidneys. A number of research studies have looked at the effect these targets have had on the long-term health of dialysis patients. All of the studies have shown that there is no benefit to exceeding the targets. Put simply, dialysis keeps people with kidney failure alive, but having more dialysis does not necessarily keep them alive for longer.

The eGFR
This test estimates the glomerular filtration rate; the rate at which blood passes through the kidneys in order for the waste products to be extracted. The eGFR is the estimated creatinine clearance of the kidneys.

It is calculated by putting the blood creatinine level into a mathematical equation. This equation makes allowances for the patient's age, gender, weight and race. In this way it 'converts' the blood creatinine level (affected by many other factors) into a percentage of normal kidney function (less affected by those factors).

At present, eGFR is mainly used in the predialysis period.

Different eGFR levels are associated with different stages of kidney failure, as shown in the table on *page 8*.

KEY FACTS

1 Creatinine and urea are two waste products that are normally passed in the urine.

2 The levels of urea and creatinine in your blood are an indication of how well the kidneys (or dialysis or a transplant) are working. Blood creatinine level is a more reliable guide than blood urea level.

3 The higher the level of urea or creatinine in your blood, the worse your kidney (dialysis or transplant) function. Generally speaking, the lower the number, the better.

4 The estimated glomerular filtration rate test or eGFR, is now being widely used, either instead of, or in addition to, creatinine clearance tests. Both are used mainly in the predialysis period.

5 The eGFR test tells the medical team how well your kidneys are working by measuring the number of millilitres of blood that are cleaned by the filtering system in your kidneys within the space of one minute. It is normally 100 mls/min, which approximates to 100% of kidney function.

6 In contrast to the blood creatinine, the lower the eGFR or creatinine clearance, the worse your kidneys (dialysis or transplant) are working. Generally speaking with this test, the higher the number, the better.

7 Ideally, dialysis should be started (or a transplant performed) when your creatinine level is 500 µmol/l, or less. At this stage, your eGFR is likely to be less than 5 mls/min (i.e. 5% function).

8 Urea and creatinine clearance tests may be more accurate ways of measuring how well your dialysis is working.

9 Kidney function continues to deteriorate after starting dialysis, making it necessary to increase the dialysis dose, usually after about one year, although this is sooner for people who have haemodialysis.

10 eGFR, blood creatinine, urea and creatinine clearance are all tests that are used to measure how well your kidneys, dialysis (or a transplant) are working. Different renal units use different methods. It is not clear yet, which is 'best'.

3 FLUID BALANCE

This chapter describes how the amount of water in the body is controlled by healthy kidneys. It looks at the problem of too much or too little water in the body when kidneys fail and gives information on how to deal with it.

INTRODUCTION

One of the two main functions of the kidneys is to remove excess water from the body. Water comes into the body from drinks, and also from food, especially high-liquid food such as soup, jelly and ice-cream. By removing excess water from the body, the kidneys are able to control the body's water content. This is called fluid balance. To understand fluid balance, it helps to know a bit about how the body is made up.

FLESH AND FLUID

The body is made up of two main parts: flesh and fluid. The flesh is all the solid parts of the body, such as bone, muscle and fat. Most of the fluid part is simply water, such as the water in blood, urine and saliva. Men have approximately 60% of fluid to 40% of flesh in their bodies, whereas women, whose bodies contain a higher proportion of fat, have approximately 55% of fluid to 45% of flesh (see *diagram*).

The easiest way to see a change in the amount of fluid in the body is to measure body weight. The known weight of 1 litre of water is 1 kilogram. So, if you weigh yourself, then drink 1 litre of water, then weigh yourself again, your weight will show an increase of 1 kilogram.

Fluid and flesh proportions in the human body

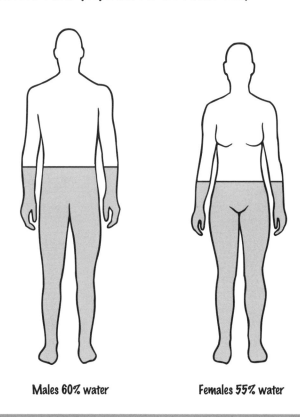

Males 60% water   Females 55% water

WHAT IS THE 'TARGET WEIGHT'?

The term 'target weight' means the weight that the doctor considers to be the 'best' weight for an individual patient. At this weight, there will be neither too much nor too little water in the body. Men will have about 60% fluid to 40% flesh, and women about 55% fluid to 45% flesh. A kidney patient's target weight may have to go up or down as flesh weight is gained or lost. Flesh weight increases if a person eats too much, or may decrease due to dieting or illness.

Weight also changes according to how much fluid is in the body. If a person has too much water in their body (i.e. is fluid overloaded, see below), they will weigh more. The target weight, therefore, is the ideal weight when the person is neither 'wet' (fluid overloaded) nor 'dry' (dehydrated). Sometimes target weight is called 'dry' weight or 'ideal' weight.

Water loss from the human body

Faeces 4%

Sweat 17%

Breath 17%

Urine 62%

Judging the amount of water in the body is difficult. But with practice, patients can learn to 'feel' when they are at their target weight.

CONTROL OF FLUID BALANCE

Normal healthy kidneys can control the amount of water in the body with ease. If you do not have kidney failure, you do not have to think about your fluid balance because your kidneys control the amount of urine you pass.

If a person drinks 10 pints of water (or beer), they will usually pass about 10 pints of urine. Similarly, if they drink three cups of tea per day, they can expect to pass the equivalent of about three tea cups of urine.

Fluid is also lost from the body in other ways – as you breathe, when you sweat and in your faeces (see diagram). If someone becomes very hot, they will sweat more. To control fluid balance, they will then need to compensate for the sweat lost by passing less urine.

In kidney failure, it is different. Many kidney patients do not pass any urine at all. Others pass exactly the same amount of urine every day, no matter how much they drink. This means these patients are unable to control how much water is in the body. If someone with kidney failure drinks too much, they may keep that fluid in their body. This is called fluid overload (see page 21 for more details). Conversely, if someone with kidney failure drinks too little, or loses too much water from the body (say, through sweating), they will become dehydrated (see page 21). Finding the balance is not always easy.

SODIUM (SALT) AND FLUID BALANCE

Sodium is a mineral that plays a part in helping to control the body's fluid balance. Too much of it can contribute to high blood pressure. Table salt contains sodium, so dialysis patients should avoid eating salty foods such as bacon, crisps and many processed foods. They should also avoid adding salt to their food either at table or in cooking. Also, eating salty foods makes people want to drink more fluid. If people with kidney failure drink too much, they may develop fluid overload.

WHAT IS FLUID OVERLOAD?

This is a condition in which there is too much water in the body. It is caused by drinking too much fluid, or not losing enough. Fluid overload also causes (or worsens) high blood pressure (see *Chapter 4*). High blood pressure may not cause any symptoms.

When the water content of the body reaches a very high level, excess water collects in and under the skin. The problem usually first shows as swelling around the ankles. This is called ankle oedema. The reason the ankles are affected first is simple – gravity tends to make fluid fall to the bottom of the body.

If fluid overload is not treated, the swelling due to excess fluid slowly creeps up the body into the thighs, and then into the lower abdomen and lower back. Hopefully, by this stage, the patient will have asked for medical help. If not, fluid will continue to spread up the body, and eventually settle in the lungs. Fluid in the lungs, which causes shortness of breath, is called pulmonary oedema. It is a very serious condition, and can be life-threatening.

Occasionally, people with kidney failure suddenly develop pulmonary oedema, without going through the 'warning stages' of ankle and leg swelling. This can happen if they drink a lot of fluid very quickly. When pulmonary oedema comes on this quickly, it needs urgent treatment. And urgent means exactly that – treatment straight away.

Fluid overload tends to occur mainly in kidney patients on dialysis. However, it can be a problem for pre-dialysis patients too, and also for people who have had a kidney transplant.

HOW IS FLUID OVERLOAD TREATED?

Remember, 'what goes in has to come out'. Therefore the first treatment of fluid overload for all people with kidney failure is simply to drink less. However, this is not usually enough. It is also important that they cut down on salt in their diet, since salt increases thirst. Additional treatments depend on whether or not the kidneys are still making urine, often referred to as having 'residual renal function (RRF)':

1. Patients with residual renal function. If patients are pre-dialysis, if they have a failing transplant, or if they are on dialysis and still pass some urine, they will usually be given tablets called diuretics 'water tablets' to treat fluid overload. The tablets work by increasing the amount of urine that is passed every day. A combination of passing more urine and drinking less usually does the trick. Two commonly used diuretic drugs are furosemide and bumetanide. Stronger diuretics, such as mefruside and metolazone, may be given as well.

If taking diuretics and drinking less does not get rid of all the fluid, it may be necessary for patients not already doing so, to have dialysis. or for patients already on dialysis to have more.

2. Patients with no residual renal function. Everyone without residual renal function requires dialysis. Dialysis patients who get fluid overload should also drink less. However, diuretics don't normally work and so a different treatment for fluid overload is needed. These patients need a combination of drinking less (usually a daily limit of 1 litre for haemodialysis patients and 1.5 litres for PD patients), and removing more water by dialysis.

DEHYDRATION

Dehydration is the opposite of fluid overload. It occurs when there is too little water in the body. Dehydration may occur if someone does not drink enough, or if they lose fluid as a result of sweating, diarrhoea or vomiting.

It can be difficult for people to judge when they are dehydrated. However, dehydration is almost always accompanied by low blood pressure. This is easier to identify than high blood pressure. Low blood pressure makes people feel weak and dizzy when they stand up.

HOW IS DEHYDRATION TREATED?

Any patient with kidney failure who is suffering from dehydration needs to drink more.

If a patient (pre-dialysis or with a failing transplant) takes diuretics, these should be reduced or stopped. If the dehydration is severe, admission to hospital for intravenous fluids (via a drip) may be necessary.

For dialysis patients, a reduction in the amount of water removed by dialysis may be needed. If haemodialysis patients are severely dehydrated, they can be given a lot of intravenous fluid during a dialysis session.

TAKING CONTROL OF YOUR OWN FLUID BALANCE

Keeping the right balance of fluid in your body is crucial for long-term health when you are on dialysis. This is particularly important if you have haemodialysis as the dialysis is not done every day and body fluid will build up between treatments.

Keeping the right balance means making sure that the amount you drink is no more than the amount of fluid that is removed by dialysis. You are in control of how much you drink, and can learn to judge how much is safe for you. You can help yourself by not eating salt or salty food, using a small cup to drink out of and spreading your drinks throughout the day. If you get thirsty, sucking an ice cube may help (but don't forget this is water too).

KEY FACTS

1 Fluid balance is the balance between water coming into the body, from drinks and food, and water leaving the body, mainly in the urine or by dialysis.

2 Too much water in the body is called fluid overload. This may cause swelling of the ankles.

3 If you eat salty foods, such as bacon, crisps and many pre-packed foods, you will become very thirsty and will not be able to control your fluid intake. So control of salt intake is vital for control of fluid intake.

4 The treatment of fluid overload is to drink less, and to remove more fluid from the body. This is done by taking diuretics (water tablets), or by increasing the amount of water removed by dialysis.

5 If fluid overload is not treated, shortness of breath due to fluid in the lungs may develop. This condition – known as pulmonary oedema – needs urgent treatment in hospital.

6 Judging the amount of water in the body is difficult. But, with practice, patients can learn to 'feel' when they are on their target weight – i.e. when they are neither 'wet' (fluid overloaded) nor 'dry' (dehydrated).

7 When there is too little water in the body (dehydration), dizziness may occur.

8 The treatment of dehydration is to drink more, and to remove less water from the body. This is done either by stopping diuretics, or by reducing the amount of water removed by dialysis.

9 Fluid balance is one area where you can really take control and do a lot to help yourself. Make sure that the amount you drink is no more than the amount of fluid that can be removed by dialysis, and learn to judge how much is safe for you. Help yourself by avoiding salty food (that makes you thirsty), using a small cup to drink out of and spreading your drinks throughout the day.

4 BLOOD PRESSURE

This chapter looks at the link between blood pressure and kidney failure. It also explains the importance of blood pressure control and how this is achieved.

INTRODUCTION

The control of blood pressure is one of the important 'extra' functions performed by the kidneys. The term 'blood pressure' means the pressure of the blood on the artery walls. This pressure goes up and down as the heart continuously squeezes and relaxes to pump blood around the body. Although the kidneys are known to help control the blood pressure, exactly how they do this is not clearly understood.

HIGH BLOOD PRESSURE AND KIDNEY FAILURE

High blood pressure is very common in people with kidney failure. The connection between these two conditions is two-way. High blood pressure can cause kidney failure, and kidney failure causes high blood pressure. It is often difficult to know for certain whether a patient's high blood pressure has caused their kidney failure, or whether kidney failure has caused their high blood pressure.

High blood pressure can occur in kidney patients who are pre-dialysis, who are on dialysis, or who have had a transplant. Many patients with kidney failure are taking one, two or even three types of blood pressure tablet.

Many patients with kidney failure have to take an injection treatment called erythropoietin stimulating agent (ESA) for anaemia. If you have high blood pressure, this treatment can make it worse. It is better, however, to stay on the drug if you need it, and to take more blood pressure tablets, than to stop ESA treatment.

LOW BLOOD PRESSURE AND KIDNEY FAILURE

Some people with kidney failure have a different blood pressure problem. Their blood pressure is lower than it should be. Low blood pressure is usually less serious than high blood pressure, but it also needs to be treated.

Very low blood pressure can be serious though. It can be a sign that the heart is not pumping well (heart failure), or fluid in the sac around the heart (pericardial effusion). Both can be treated.

CIRCULATION OF THE BLOOD

The main function of the blood (and the blood vessels through which it flows) is to carry things around the body. Blood carries 'good things' to parts of the body where they are needed, and also removes 'bad things' so they can be got rid of, mainly by the kidneys via the urine.

Adults have about 5 litres (10 pints) of blood travelling around their body all the time. The heart acts as a pump to drive the blood through the blood vessels. There are two main types of blood vessel: arteries and veins. The arteries take blood that is rich in oxygen from the heart

Circulation of blood in the human body

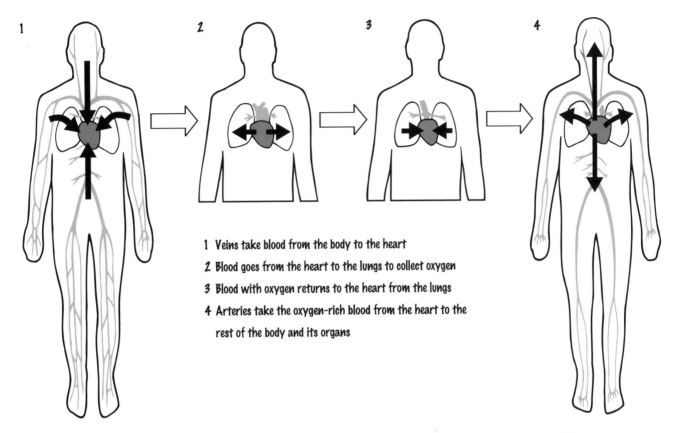

1 Veins take blood from the body to the heart

2 Blood goes from the heart to the lungs to collect oxygen

3 Blood with oxygen returns to the heart from the lungs

4 Arteries take the oxygen-rich blood from the heart to the
   rest of the body and its organs

to all parts of the body. This oxygen, combined with the food that is eaten, provides the different parts of the body with the energy they need to do their work. The veins then take the blood (now with most of its oxygen used up) back to the heart. From there, the blood goes to the lungs to get more oxygen. It then goes back to the heart, and so the process goes on (see *diagram* above).

MEASURING BLOOD PRESSURE

The blood pressure is measured using a piece of equipment known as a sphygmomanometer (or sphyg,

pronounced 'sfig'). There are various different types of sphygmomanometer, but all of them measure blood pressure in units of millimetres of mercury (mmHg).

Two readings are taken. The first reading shows the pressure of the blood when the heart squeezes, and is called the systolic blood pressure. The second reading is the pressure of the blood when the heart is relaxed between squeezes. This is called the diastolic blood pressure.

The systolic pressure is always higher than the diastolic pressure, and is always recorded first. So, for example, a blood pressure of 130/80 mmHg (known

Blood pressure

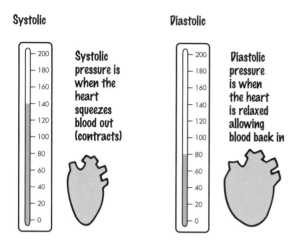

Systolic

Systolic pressure is when the heart squeezes blood out (contracts)

Diastolic

Diastolic pressure is when the heart is relaxed allowing blood back in

For most people with kidney failure, however, doctors accept a level of 130/80 or below as satisfactory. This is for patients who are not yet on dialysis, those on PD or with a transplant, or before a haemodialysis session.

The blood pressure varies continuously throughout the heart's pumping cycle. This means that during each cycle, the systolic blood pressure is, say, 140 or 180 for only a fraction of a second.

Blood pressure also varies according to the time of day – tending to be higher in the morning and again in the early evening. And there is a difference between one arm and the other. Slight variations may also result from using different sphygmomanometers, or from how different people use the same piece of equipment.

If there is doubt about whether or not a patient has high blood pressure, a 24-hour blood pressure test can be organised. This involves a patient carrying a cuff on their arm for 24 hours. Every hour, the cuff automatically inflates and deflates, giving the doctor a better idea of the average blood pressure over the 24-hour period.

as '130 over 80') means that the systolic pressure is 130 and the diastolic pressure is 80.

A reading of 130 mmHg means that the blood pressure has raised the top of the mercury (Hg) column inside the sphygmomanometer to a height of 130 millimetres.

WHAT IS 'NORMAL' BLOOD PRESSURE?

There is no such thing as normal blood pressure. Both the systolic and the diastolic blood pressure go up naturally as people get older. So there is only a normal *range* of blood pressure for your age. Most doctors accept the following values as the normal range for different age groups:

Age Group	Blood Pressure (in mmHg)	
	Systolic	**Diastolic**
Under 30 years	100–120	60–70
30–60 years	110–130	70–80
Over 60 years	120–140	80–90

DOES ANXIETY AFFECT BLOOD PRESSURE?

Anxiety is definitely not a major factor in high blood pressure. Although anxiety can put the blood pressure up a little, it is a mistake to blame repeated high blood pressure readings on, for example, 'the stress of the journey' or a 'fear of seeing the doctor', or even 'difficulty parking'.

HOW DO YOU KNOW THAT YOUR BLOOD PRESSURE IS HIGH OR LOW?

You don't. Some people with very high blood pressure suffer from headaches. But the fact that you do not have headaches does not mean that you do not have high blood pressure. The only reliable way of finding out what your blood pressure is, is to have it measured.

If your blood pressure is very low, you may feel weak or dizzy, especially when you stand up. But there are many other causes of weakness and dizziness. So, as with high blood pressure, you cannot rely on your body to tell you that your blood pressure is low. You have to have your blood pressure checked.

WHY TREAT HIGH BLOOD PRESSURE?

There are several important reasons to treat high blood pressure. However, there is little point in treating someone for high blood pressure unless the related problems of high cholesterol levels in the blood, being overweight and smoking are also addressed. All these factors worsen the effects of high blood pressure.

High blood pressure increases the likelihood of a stroke or a heart attack by damaging the blood vessels. There are also 'kidney reasons' to treat high blood pressure. If blood pressure is high for a period of time, a patient with kidney failure may have to start dialysis sooner than would otherwise be necessary. This is because uncontrolled high blood pressure can accelerate kidney failure.

In fact, controlling blood pressure is the only thing proven to delay the need for dialysis in all kidney patients, whatever the cause of their kidney failure. Good blood pressure control does not mean they will never need dialysis, but it may mean that dialysis does not need to be started so soon. It may also prolong the life of a transplant.

WHAT DETERMINES BLOOD PRESSURE LEVELS?

A person's blood pressure is affected by the following important factors:

1. The amount of water in the body. If there is too much water in the body (fluid overload), the blood pressure will go up. If there is too little water in the body (dehydration), the blood pressure will go down. (Both fluid overload and dehydration, and their treatments, are described in *Chapter 3*.)

2. The width of the arteries. The arteries are constantly changing in width as blood flows through them. The narrower the arteries, the higher the blood pressure.

3. The heart (the pump). The strength of contraction of the heart, and the rate it beats, also affect blood pressure. Generally speaking, the harder or faster the heart beats, the higher the blood pressure will be.

HOW IS HIGH BLOOD PRESSURE TREATED?

Because there are 3 main factors contributing to high blood pressure, there are also 3 different ways of treating it:

1. By reducing the amount of water in the body. If someone has fluid overload, their blood pressure will increase. This is because their blood contains more water than normal, which increases the pressure on the blood vessels. Correcting fluid overload (see *Chapter 3*) with diuretics (water tablets) or dialysis will reduce the blood pressure. Eating a lot of salty foods and adding extra salt to meals makes people thirsty and leads to them drinking more (see *page 21*). So people with kidney failure should cut down on salt as well as fluid.

2. By increasing the width of the arteries (with vasodilator drugs). Blood pressure tablets called vasodilators lower the blood pressure by causing the arteries to widen. There are several different types of vasodilator drug:

- ACE inhibitors (e.g. captopril, enalapril, lisinopril, perindopril and ramipril);

- alphablockers (e.g. doxazosin, prazosin and terazosin);

- calcium antagonists (e.g. amlodipine, diltiazem, felodipine and nifedipine);

- ARBs (e.g. candesartan, irbesartan, losartan, telmisartan); and

- other tablets (e.g. hydralazine, methyldopa, minoxidil and moxonidine). Minoxidil is probably the strongest drug available, and can be extremely useful for kidney patients with very high blood pressure.

3. By decreasing the strength of contraction of the heart, and the rate at which it beats (using beta-blocker drugs). These tablets reduce the force of contraction and the heart rate (the number of heart beats per minute). They also lower the blood pressure, although how they do this is not clear. Commonly used examples of beta-blockers are atenolol, bisoprolol, carvedilol, labetalol, metoprolol and propranolol.

ARE THE BLOOD PRESSURE TABLETS WORKING?

As blood pressure has to be very high before it causes symptoms (such as headaches), most people cannot 'feel' that their blood pressure is raised. Not surprisingly, therefore, they also cannot tell whether or not their blood pressure tablets are working. The only reliable way of knowing a person's blood pressure, and discovering whether it is responding to tablets, is for the blood pressure to be measured.

DOES SALT IN FOOD AFFECT BLOOD PRESSURE?

Too much sodium (salt) in the body can increase the blood pressure. This is because a salty diet makes people thirsty and encourages them to drink more. However, salt is not the only thing that causes high blood pressure (see page 27). People who have high blood pressure will be asked to eat less salt and take tablets to help keep it under control.

WHAT ABOUT LOW BLOOD PRESSURE?

Low blood pressure is not as common as high blood pressure. It is normally less serious and easier to treat. This is partly because people can often feel that their blood pressure is low. So they can also feel when it is back to normal.

Low blood pressure in people with kidney failure is usually due either to dehydration, or to taking too many blood pressure tablets. Therefore, the treatment is either to drink more to correct the dehydration, or to alter the dose of blood pressure tablets or stop the tablets.

TAKING CONTROL OF YOUR OWN BLOOD PRESSURE

High blood pressure is not something you just need to 'suffer' with. The three golden rules for keeping your blood pressure down are:

- take your blood pressure tablets;

- don't get fluid-overloaded;

- don't eat too much salt.

KEY FACTS

1 High blood pressure is very common in people with kidney failure.

2 An acceptable blood pressure will be 130/80 or below, for most people.

3 Kidney failure causes high blood pressure, and high blood pressure causes kidney failure.

4 The injection treatment for anaemia, called erythropoietin stimulating agents (ESAs), can increase your blood pressure.

5 High blood pressure also increases the likelihood of a stroke or heart attack.

6 You cannot reliably 'feel' your own blood pressure, especially when it is high. You have to have it checked.

7 High blood pressure can be controlled by removing fluid from your body and by taking blood pressure tablets.

8 Too much salt in the diet may make the blood pressure higher.

9 You have the opportunity to take a large part of responsibility for controlling your own blood pressure. Have it checked regularly, don't drink too much fluid, avoid salt wherever possible, and make sure you take the tablets your doctor prescribes for you.

5 ANAEMIA AND ERYTHROPOIETIN

This chapter explains what anaemia is, and how erythropoietin stimulating agents (ESAs) have revolutionised its treatment. ESAs are probably the most important drugs taken by patients who need them.

INTRODUCTION

Many patients with kidney failure have a condition called anaemia. This means that they have a lack of red blood cells in their body. Blood cells are produced in the bone marrow, the 'runny' bit in the middle of the bones. An important 'extra' function of the kidneys is to help control the manufacture of red blood cells in the bone marrow.

WHAT IS ANAEMIA?

Anaemia is the term for a lack of red blood cells in the body. The main symptoms are tiredness, shortness of breath, pale skin, poor appetite, irritability and low sex drive. Anaemia is probably the most important complication of kidney failure. It is the main reason why dialysis patients feel weak and tired. In fact, many of the symptoms of kidney failure are not caused by kidney failure itself, but are actually due to anaemia.

Red blood cells are needed to carry oxygen around the body. Oxygen enters the lungs when we breathe in. From the lungs, oxygen is taken around the body in the blood. Each red blood cell contains a substance called haemoglobin. It is the haemoglobin that carries oxygen around the body. Oxygen combines with the nutrients taken in from food to provide energy.

Location of bone marrow

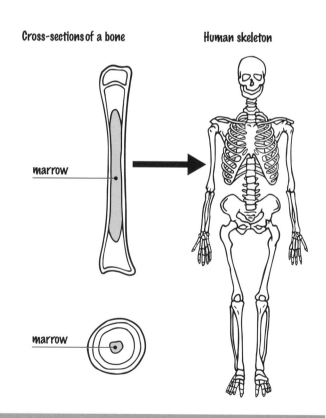

Cross-sections of a bone

Human skeleton

marrow

marrow

Measuring the level of haemoglobin (or 'Hb') in the blood provides a guide to the number of red cells present. The higher the Hb, the more red blood cells there are in the body. As it is red blood cells that are able to carry oxygen round the body, in general the higher the Hb the better (but see *page 32*).

Normal Hb levels are 12–17 g/dl (grams of haemoglobin per decilitre of blood).

- **If your Hb is below 11 g/dl, you have anaemia**.

COMPOSITION OF THE BLOOD

Blood is made up of two parts: a liquid part and a more solid part. The liquid part is called plasma. It accounts for about 60% of the blood's volume, and is mainly water. The amount of water in the plasma is increased in fluid overload and decreased in dehydration. (Both these conditions were described in *Chapter 3*.)

The other 40% of the blood is made up of blood cells, which are so tiny that they can only be seen through a microscope. There are various different types of cells: red cells (which carry oxygen around the body), white cells (which fight infection) and platelets (involved in blood clotting). Most of the blood cells are red cells. It is these cells that give the blood its red colour. Each one looks rather like a tiny doughnut. Red cells are smaller than white cells, and larger than platelets. You have about 5 billion red cells in one drop of blood.

WHY DO PEOPLE WITH KIDNEY FAILURE DEVELOP ANAEMIA?

The main reason that kidney patients develop anaemia is this. One of the jobs the kidneys do, in addition to their main job of making urine, is to manage the production of red blood cells in the bone marrow. To do this, the kidneys make a substance called erythropoietin (EPO).

EPO travels in the blood from the kidneys to the bone

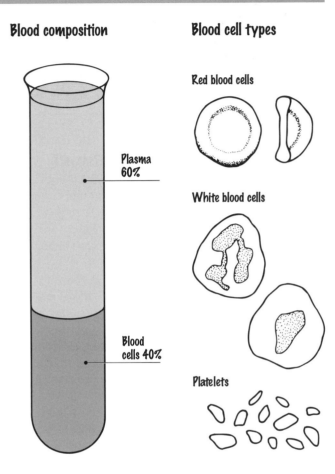

Blood composition

Plasma 60%

Blood cells 40%

Blood cell types

Red blood cells

White blood cells

Platelets

marrow, where it constantly reminds the bone marrow to keep producing red cells. When someone has kidney failure, the kidneys usually make less EPO than normal. So the bone marrow 'goes to sleep' and makes fewer red cells. As a result, anaemia develops, and the patient becomes weak and tired.

Some patients with kidney failure develop anaemia even though their EPO level is normal (or even high). This probably means that their bone marrow has a problem reacting to EPO, rather than that the kidneys are not making enough EPO. Although a lack of EPO is the main cause of anaemia in people with kidney failure, other things may contribute. For example, red blood cells do not live as long as normal (120 days) in people with kidney failure, and so must be replaced more rapidly. Also, blood may be lost during haemodialysis, or through frequent blood tests.

PROBLEMS WITH BLOOD TRANSFUSIONS

In the past – before the introduction of EPO Stimulating Agent (ESA) injections (see below) – blood transfusions were the only treatment for anaemia in kidney patients. Many patients had to have transfusions every couple of months, since each transfusion could improve anaemia for a few weeks only.

Blood transfusions can cause serious problems for patients on dialysis. These include fluid overload (see Chapter 3), and the storage of surplus iron in the liver (which can lead to liver failure). Another problem is that whenever a transfusion of blood is received, the body produces substances called antibodies. These antibodies stay in the blood for years and can cause problems if the patient is then given a transplant. The antibodies can attack (and cause the body to reject) the new kidney.

The risk of contracting hepatitis B, hepatitis C or HIV (the virus that causes AIDS) from a blood transfusion is small in the UK. Even so, if someone does not need a blood transfusion, it is better not to have one.

Blood transfusions are still sometimes needed by kidney patients – for example, after severe bleeding. In general, however, treatment with ESAs has turned regular blood transfusions into a thing of the past for kidney patients.

ESA – THE 'WONDER DRUG'

Synthetically produced ESAs became available as an injection in the late 1980s – probably the most important advance in the treatment of patients with kidney failure. In 2007, 92% of haemodialysis patients and 74% of PD patients were on an ESA. This is because patients on PD tend to have less of a problem with anaemia. If they are prescribed an ESA, they usually need a lower dose.

ESAs work well in most patients, and usually get rid of the tiredness and other symptoms caused by anaemia.

An ESA is generally given in the form of an injection under the skin (called a subcutaneous injection). This is needed one to three times a week, though there are now newer forms of ESA such as darbepoetin alfa (Aranesp) which can be given less frequently than traditional ESAs (sometimes every 2 weeks). Some patients may be asked to give their own injections, particularly those on home dialysis such as PD. The aim of the treatment is to raise the Hb level in the blood to between 11 and 12 g/dl. Without this treatment, most patients with kidney failure will have an Hb between 6 and 8 g/dl.

A patient's response to an ESA depends on how much they are given. The higher or more frequent the dose, the higher the patient's blood Hb level will go. However, there is no point in making the Hb go above 12 g/dl – the patient will feel no better. In fact, problems may occur if the Hb goes over 14 g/dl. For example, a fistula may clot and stop working. So, the target Hb is 11–12 g/dl in most patients, and they should take ESAs only as prescribed.

WHO NEEDS AN ESA?

Patients who are on dialysis – either PD (see Chapter 9) or haemodialysis (see Chapter 10) – often need an ESA. But, for most patients, anaemia actually begins long before they need to start dialysis. Therefore many doctors now give ESAs before the start of dialysis, in the predialysis period. Transplant patients should also be considered for an ESA if their Hb falls below 11 g/dl, especially if the transplant is failing, as anaemia often returns at this time. However, there are some doctors who prefer to delay starting treatment with an ESA until 3 months after the start of dialysis. This is because the start of dialysis will sometimes 'cure' a patient's anaemia – perhaps because dialysis removes toxins that may interfere with the way the bone marrow works.

Treatment with ESAs has been found to be very useful even in those kidney failure patients who have anaemia without having a reduced EPO level. It is not known why giving very high doses of an ESA to these patients should make such a difference to their anaemia, but it does.

Some patients with kidney failure – especially those with polycystic kidney disease (see page 6) – do not become anaemic, as their kidneys continue to produce EPO, even when on dialysis. They therefore do not usually need ESA treatment.

ARE THERE ANY SIDE EFFECTS?

The only common side effect of ESAs is worsening of high blood pressure. This is most likely in patients who have had severe high blood pressure in the past, or in patients who are on more than one type of blood pressure tablet. If the blood pressure does increase, more blood pressure tablets may need to be taken. A combination of an ESA and high blood pressure can sometimes cause epileptic fits, but this problem can usually be prevented by treating the high blood pressure.

POOR RESPONSE TO ESA TREATMENT

Most, but not all, patients respond to regular treatment with ESAs. However, an ESA may not work if other conditions are present. These include infections – especially repeated peritonitis PD patients, and dialysis catheter site infections in haemodialysis patients. It also may not work if there is under-dialysis (failure of dialysis to achieve target creatinine and urea levels),

renal bone disease (see Chapter 6) or iron deficiency.

Iron deficiency is the most common reason for an ESA not to work. ESAs cause the body's iron stores to be used up more quickly than usual. In an attempt to spot the onset of iron deficiency, patients are given regular blood tests to measure a substance called ferritin (see page 46). Blood ferritin levels provide a guide to the amount of iron stored in the body and low levels of ferritin indicate iron deficiency. So, generally speaking, higher ferritin levels are better. The value should be at least 200 micrograms per litre.

If iron deficiency is discovered, the doctors should investigate why the patient lacks iron. One important cause could be bleeding (that may not have been noticed by the patient) from somewhere in the bowel.

If such causes of iron deficiency can be ruled out, it can sometimes be treated with iron tablets (usually a type called ferrous sulphate). Other patients need regular iron injections. These days, iron injections rather than tablets are usually given.

If an ESA stops working – for whatever reason – the Hb will return to the 'normal' low level in people with kidney failure (usually 6–8 g/dl). The symptoms of anaemia will then return.

ANAEMIA AND TRANSPLANTATION

After a kidney transplant, the new kidney will start making EPO for the patient and the problem of anaemia usually goes away. Injections of an ESA will then no longer be needed. However, if the transplanted kidney ever fails, anaemia will usually return, and ESA injections may be needed again.

KEY FACTS

1 Many patients who have kidney failure (predialysis, on dialysis or with a transplant) have a condition called anaemia. This means you have a lack of red blood cells.

2 Anaemia is the main reason why dialysis patients are weak and tired.

3 The severity of anaemia is measured by a blood test called a haemoglobin (or 'Hb') test.

4 If your Hb is below 11 g/dl, you have anaemia.

5 The lower your Hb level, the more anaemic and tired you will be.

6 Anaemia is easy to treat with injections of substances called erythropoietin stimulating agents (ESAs). Examples include epoetin (e.g. NeoRecormon or Eprex) and darbepoetin alfa (Aranesp).

7 All patients (predialysis, on dialysis or with a transplant) with an Hb below 11 g/dl should be considered for an ESA. The target Hb is 11–12 g/dl in most patients. Ferritin levels should be kept above 200 µg/L.

8 Patients on ESA treatment may need additional iron in the form of either tablets or injections.

9 ESAs are very good at controlling symptoms and giving you more energy. You should only stop taking them or miss a dose if your kidney doctor tells you to.

10 If you have a transplant that is working well, you can usually stop taking an ESA.

6 RENAL BONE DISEASE

This chapter provides information on the causes, prevention and treatment of renal bone disease (also known as renal osteo-dystrophy), which is a common problem for people with kidney failure.

INTRODUCTION

Most people with kidney failure have some degree of renal bone disease. This is because one of the 'extra' functions of the kidneys is to help make the bones strong and healthy. For the bones to be strong, the kidneys must be able to maintain a healthy balance of various substances – including calcium, phosphate and vitamin D – in the body. Kidney failure results in abnormal levels of these substances, and so leads to renal bone disease.

DEVELOPMENT OF RENAL BONE DISEASE

Blood tests will reveal abnormal levels of calcium, phosphate and vitamin D in a patient's blood very early in kidney failure, long before dialysis is required. The calcium and vitamin D levels will be lower than they should be, while the phosphate level will be too high. These changes can be seen in Stage 2 of chronic kidney failure (i.e. 60–90% kidney function).

Abnormalities in calcium, phosphate and vitamin D levels do not usually lead to problems that a patient is likely to notice until after the start of dialysis. However, treatment should be started at an early stage to prevent weakening of the bones. This may also help prevent problems with the heart.

WHAT DOES RENAL BONE DISEASE DO?

Without treatment, renal bone disease can lead to pain in the bones, especially in the back, hips, legs and knees. The weakened bones also become increasingly prone to fracture. The heart can also be affected. However, early recognition and treatment of renal bone disease means that bone pain and fractures are now uncommon in kidney patients.

WHAT CAUSES RENAL BONE DISEASE?

There are three main causes of renal bone disease:

1. Low calcium levels in the blood. Calcium is a mineral that strengthens the bones. It is obtained from some foods, especially dairy products, eggs and green vegetables. In our bodies, calcium is stored in the bones. There is also some calcium in the blood. The kidneys normally help to keep calcium in the bones. In people with kidney failure, calcium drains out of the bones and is lost from the body. This leads to a fall in the level of calcium in the blood.

The normal blood calcium level is between 2.1 and 2.6 mmol/l (millimoles per litre of blood). In kidney patients, the level of calcium in the blood may fall below 2.0 mmol/l. Treatment can keep the calcium level up quite easily.

2. High phosphate levels in the blood. Phosphate is another mineral that strengthens the bones. Foods that contain phosphate include dairy products, nuts and meat. Like calcium, phosphate is stored in the body in the bones and is also present in the blood. The kidneys normally help to keep the right amount in the blood – not too much, not too little. In people with kidney failure, phosphate builds up in the blood.

The normal level of phosphate in the blood is 0.75–1.4 mmol/l. In kidney patients, it is common for the blood phosphate level to be high, rising to more than 2.0 mmol/l. Unfortunately, it is quite difficult to keep phosphate levels normal. High phosphate levels are thought to cause itching.

3. Low vitamin D levels in the blood. Vitamin D is needed in the body so that calcium from the diet can be absorbed into the body and used to strengthen the bones. Vitamin D is found in some foods, especially margarine and butter. However, most of our vitamin D is made by the skin (a process that only occurs if the skin is stimulated by sunlight). Unfortunately, vitamin D from food and from the skin are in a form which the body cannot use directly. The kidneys are responsible for transforming vitamin D into a usable substance.

Blood levels of the usable form of vitamin D are not usually measured, as the blood test is expensive and difficult to do. If they were measured, they would be low. It is quite easy to provide additional vitamin D as tablets or injections, although not all kidney patients need it. Often, it will be enough just to control the levels of calcium and phosphate.

A COMBINATION OF CAUSES

Doctors do not know which of the three main causes of renal bone disease comes first. Nor do they know what leads to what. They do know, however, that although any one of these causes can lead to problems, a combination of the three is usually present in people with kidney failure. More importantly, each of the causes tends to have a 'knock-on' effect, worsening the other two abnormalities. For example, a high phosphate level tends to lower the calcium level, and vice versa. It is important, therefore, to treat all three causes (see *page 37*).

PARATHYROID HORMONE AND KIDNEY FAILURE

Parathyroid hormone (PTH) is a substance produced by four tiny glands called the parathyroid glands. These glands are situated in the front of the neck (see *diagram*). Normally the parathyroid glands (and the kidney) keep calcium, phosphate and vitamin D levels in balance. When someone has kidney failure, however, the parathyroid glands become overactive and produce too much PTH, and renal bone disease starts.

Location of the parathyroid glands

The parathyroid glands (a) are four tiny glands located at the back of the thyroid gland (b), in the neck

HOW IS RENAL BONE DISEASE MONITORED?

The levels of calcium and phosphate in a kidney patient's blood can tell us what is happening in the bones at the time of the test. However, these levels provide little information about the future.

The best guide to the progress and severity of renal bone disease is the amount of PTH in the blood. PTH tells us much more about the long-term health of the bones. Changes in blood PTH can tell us about what will happen to the bones in the future – the lower the PTH, the better.

Renal bone disease begins very early in kidney failure. It is therefore a good idea for doctors to measure a patient's blood PTH even before treatment with dialysis or a transplant is necessary. Once dialysis has started, most doctors should measure the blood PTH at least every 3 months. A high level (i.e. greater than 20 picomoles per litre of fluid) indicates a problem with the bones. Doctors will then start a range of treatments to help prevent any worsening of the problem. Even very high PTH levels can usually be lowered with the right tablets.

The target PTH level is less than twice the upper limit of normal (normal is 1.1–4.2 pmol/l). So a PTH level of less than 10 pmol/l is considered satisfactory.

HOW IS RENAL BONE DISEASE TREATED?

Treatment may be needed for each of the three main causes of renal bone disease. All patients with kidney failure, whether they are predialysis, on dialysis or with a transplant, have some degree of renal bone disease. Most will require treatment.

1. Raising low calcium levels. Patients on dialysis can obtain some extra calcium from the dialysis fluid. This happens because there is more calcium in some dialysis fluids than there is in the blood. Calcium passes from the stronger solution (the dialysis fluid) into the patient's blood (the weaker solution) by a process called diffusion. (See *Chapter 8* for more information on diffusion.)

For many kidney patients, extra calcium from dialysis is not enough. They also need calcium in the form of a drug. One commonly used form of calcium is calcium carbonate (usually taken in a preparation called Calcichew). Some renal units use another similar preparation called calcium acetate. Calcium tablets may need to be taken every day to look after the long-term health of the bones.

Although the main job of calcium in kidney patients is to reduce blood phosphate levels (see *below, point 2*), it also has the effect of raising blood calcium levels. Blood calcium levels are also raised by treatment with vitamin D (see *page 38, point 3*).

Treatment is most successful when blood calcium levels are driven to the upper end of normal. So the target blood calcium level for someone with kidney failure should be 2.4–2.5 mmol/l (given the normal range of 2.1–2.6 mmol/l).

2. Lowering high phosphate levels. Dialysis removes some phosphate from the blood, but it does not do this very efficiently. Most patients therefore need further treatment to control the phosphate level.

To lower their blood phosphate levels, kidney patients are usually given tablets called phosphate binders. The most commonly used phosphate binder is calcium (see *above, point 1*). Aluminium hydroxide used to be given as a phosphate binder too, but is rarely used these days because of the toxic effects of aluminium. Other newer drugs including sevelamer and lanthanum (alternatives to calcium) are now being offered to some patients. To be effective, any type of phosphate binder needs to be taken just before food, and not at the same time as iron tablets.

If the combination of dialysis and phosphate-binding tablets fails to control a patient's phosphate level, then it will be necessary for the patient to have more dialysis, or to eat fewer high-phosphate foods (see *Chapter 14, page 106*), or both of these.

Even with treatment, a kidney patient's blood phosphate level rarely returns to the normal level of 0.75–1.4 mmol/l. So the target blood phosphate level is not normal: it is a level of less than 1.8 mmol/l, and preferably less than 1.6 mmol/l. This target applies all the time for a PD patient, and before dialysis for a haemodialysis patient. This is difficult to achieve.

3. Raising low vitamin D levels. In a few patients, renal bone disease continues to be a problem even when the blood calcium and phosphate levels are brought under control. Treatment with a vitamin D preparation is then needed. The most commonly used type is called alfacalcidol. Another newer drug is called paricalcitol.

Vitamin D treatment works in two ways: it provides the vitamin D that is lacking and it increases blood calcium levels (see a*bove, point 1*). PD patients receive vitamin D in the form of a tablet. Haemodialysis patients receive it either as tablet, or as an injection given during dialysis.

PARATHYROIDECTOMY

In most patients, correcting the blood levels of calcium, phosphate and vitamin D is enough to control renal bone disease, and cause PTH levels to fall.

In a few patients, however, this treatment plan is not sufficient, and blood PTH levels continue to rise – especially if the blood PTH level is over 100 pmol/l and not falling (the target level is below 10 pmol/1). When this happens, the blood calcium tends to rise to above normal (it is usually low in kidney failure). At this stage, the blood phosphate is usually very high. This combination of an extremely high PTH, a high calcium and a very high phosphate level cannot be treated by dialysis and tablets alone. An operation to remove the parathyroid glands will be needed. This operation is called a parathyroidectomy.

If an operation is not performed, the blood vessels (especially those that supply blood to the heart) can become 'furred up' with calcium, which can be very dangerous. Calcium may also be deposited in the eyes (making them red and itchy) or in the skin (which can cause parts of the skin to go black and die). A parathyroidectomy is a very effective operation. It returns blood calcium levels to normal, and can prevent these complications.

A parathyroidectomy operation takes 1–2 hours, and requires a hospital stay of 5–7 days after the operation. For the next few weeks, frequent blood calcium checks will be needed. This is because blood calcium can fall to a very low level after the operation. It is often necessary for patients to take high doses of calcium carbonate and/or vitamin D after a parathyroidectomy. These can usually be stopped at a later date.

A new drug called cinacalcet can be used in some patients as an alternative to parathyroidectomy.

TRANSPLANTS AND RENAL BONE DISEASE

If a patient receives a transplant and the new kidney works well, the blood levels of calcium, phosphate, vitamin D and PTH will usually return to normal, or near normal. Renal bone disease then improves, although it never really goes away completely.

If a transplanted kidney never functions properly, or if it starts to fail after working well, renal bone disease will become a problem. It is therefore important to pay attention to the calcium, phosphate and PTH levels even after a transplant.

BONE PAIN DUE TO DIALYSIS AMYLOIDOSIS

Renal bone disease is not the only cause of bone pain in patients with kidney failure. Bone pain can also be caused by a condition called dialysis amyloidosis.

This condition develops 10 years or so after the start of kidney failure. It is caused by a poor removal by dialysis of a protein called amyloid. This causes a build-up of amyloid in the body, which continues even when a patient starts dialysis. After a time, amyloid is deposited in the joints all over the body, especially in the wrists and shoulders. This leads to joint and bone pain.

At present, there is no effective treatment for this condition in dialysis patients. Its progress is halted – to an extent – by transplantation.

KEY FACTS

1 Renal bone disease is an important complication of kidney failure.

2 Without treatment, renal bone disease can cause bone pain and fractures, and may also affect your heart.

3 All patients with kidney failure, whether they are predialysis, on dialysis or have a transplant, have some degree of renal bone disease. Most will need treatment.

4 Renal bone disease is caused by low levels of calcium and vitamin D in the blood, and by high blood levels of phosphate.

5 A combination of tablets usually reverses these problems.

6 The best way of finding out how healthy your bones are in the long term, is to measure the level of parathyroid hormone (PTH) in your blood. The higher the PTH level, the worse your bones. A level of 10 pmol/l or below is OK.

7 If the doctors cannot control your renal bone disease, you may need an operation called a parathyroidectomy to remove the parathyroid glands in your neck.

7 BLOOD TESTS AND OTHER TESTS

Blood tests are very important in kidney failure. They are one of the best ways of telling how well dialysis or a transplant is working. The information in this chapter will help you to understand the results of your tests.

INTRODUCTION

The majority of this chapter is concerned with blood tests, but other tests that patients may experience during the course of kidney failure will be explained in the later sections. Although the chapter is written mainly for patients on dialysis, the general principles described are also true for patients who have not yet started dialysis, or who have had a kidney transplant.

All patients with kidney failure have regular blood tests. Blood test results provide doctors and nurses with the information they need to treat their kidney patients as effectively as possible. Patients who learn to understand their own blood test results can find out a lot about what is going on inside their body. They can also assess for themselves how well their treatment is working.

THE 'FIGURES'

The term 'figures' is commonly used in hospitals to refer to the biochemistry blood test that most kidney patients have at the end of every clinic appointment. It is important to understand that every hospital will be using different measuring equipment and there will be some variation in what are considered 'normal' values

throughout the UK. So don't assume you must have the same values as someone who attends a hospital 50 miles away. Also, hospitals occasionally change their 'normal' ranges. In addition, there may be differences in the normal ranges given for men and for women. The figures given in this chapter represent an average range, but do check what range is considered normal, for men and for women, at your hospital.

The biochemistry blood test is not really a single test. It includes measurements of a whole range of different substances in the blood. Most patients with kidney failure tend to focus on two of them: creatinine and potassium. This is a good choice, as they are probably the two most important tests. Both of them indicate how well dialysis is working.

However, looking at blood test results can give you a lot of information about your body. You (and the doctors) can gain information about the levels of minerals in your body, the acidity of your blood, the state of your bones, how well nourished you are, and how well your liver is working.

The dozen or so substances usually measured in a biochemistry blood test for kidney patients can be divided into two groups: dialysable and non-dialysable (i.e. those that are affected by dialysis, and those that are not).

TESTS FOR DIALYSABLE SUBSTANCES

The first group of substances measured in the biochemistry blood test for kidney patients are all dialysable. This means that they can pass from the blood into the dialysis solution, and vice versa. The direction in which a dialysable substance travels during dialysis depends on the amount of substance in the blood and in the dialysis solution. Substances always pass – by a process called diffusion – from a stronger to a weaker solution. (See *Chapter 8* for a more detailed description of this basic principle of dialysis.)

By putting more or less of different substances in the dialysis fluid, compared with the blood, it is possible to remove substances from the blood, or to add them to the body. The biochemistry test measures blood levels of several substances that may be removed from the body by dialysis – potassium, creatinine, urea and phosphate. It also measures the levels of some useful substances that are given to patients in the dialysis fluid – bicarbonate and calcium. Two other dialysable substances – sodium and glucose – are also measured, although the blood levels of these substances are not usually affected by dialysis.

1. Potassium.
The chemical symbol for potassium is K. It is a dialysable mineral that is usually present in the blood. The normal level of potassium in the blood is 3.7–5.0 mmol/l (millimoles per litre of blood). Potassium helps the heart to function properly.

Patients with kidney failure tend to have too much potassium in the blood, although there are some patients who have too little. Either too much or too little potassium can be dangerous, eventually causing the heart to stop and the patient to die. Problems are especially likely if the blood potassium is more than 7.0 mmol/l, or less than 2.0 mmol/l. These are the danger lines.

There is no potassium in peritoneal dialysis (PD) fluid, and only a small amount (usually less than 2.0 mmol/l) in haemodialysis fluid. Because of the basic principle of dialysis (by which substances pass from a stronger to a weaker solution), potassium usually flows out of the blood into the dialysis fluid. Dialysis therefore normally removes potassium from the body.

Controlling the level of potassium in the blood can be quite difficult, especially in patients who are being treated by haemodialysis. Because of this, it may be necessary for some haemodialysis patients to restrict their intake of potassium-rich foods in between dialysis sessions. However, because PD is a continuous treatment, patients who are on PD will not usually find it quite so difficult to control their potassium levels (see also *Chapter 14, page 106*).

Despite the difficulties, a normal potassium level can usually be achieved.

2. Creatinine.
Creatinine is a waste substance produced by the muscles whenever they are used. Like thousands of other body wastes, creatinine is carried around the body in the blood until it is normally filtered out by the kidneys and passed in the urine (see *page 1*).

Creatinine is not in itself harmful to the body, but it is a very important 'marker', which provides a valuable guide to the levels of other, less easily measured substances in the blood. If there is a build-up of creatinine in the blood, there will also be a build-up of many other more harmful substances. The higher the creatinine level, the worse the kidney, dialysis or transplant function (see *Chapter 2* for more details).

The normal level of creatinine in the blood is 50–120 µmol/l (micromoles per litre of blood). There is no creatinine in dialysis fluid. Because creatinine is dialysable, it passes out of the blood, through the dialysis membrane (see *Chapter 8*) into the dialysis fluid.

Creatinine levels can never be normal when someone is on dialysis. This is because dialysis – whether PD or haemodialysis – can provide only about 5% of the function of two healthy kidneys.

For a patient of average size who is on PD, the target creatinine level is below 600 µmol/l. For a similar patient on haemodialysis, the target is below 600 µmol/l before dialysis, and below 250 µmol/l after dialysis. Larger, more muscular people produce more creatinine than smaller, less muscular people. Because of this, individual creatinine targets are adjusted to take account of body and muscle size. Provided this adjustment is made, the creatinine level is a very reliable guide to a patient's kidney (dialysis or transplant) function (see *Chapter 2* for more details).

3. Urea. Urea is a waste product of food. It is made in the liver and then travels in the blood to the kidneys, where it normally goes into the urine for removal from the body. Like creatinine, urea is a 'marker' for other, more harmful substances in the blood. A build-up of urea in the blood also indicates a build-up of many other substances. The higher the blood urea level, the worse is the kidney (dialysis or transplant) function (see *Chapter 2* for more details).

The normal range for urea in the blood is 2.6–6.6 mmol/l. There is no urea in dialysis fluid. Again, because urea is dialysable, it will pass out of the blood into the dialysis fluid. Urea levels can never be normal when someone is on dialysis. Neither type of dialysis is good enough at getting rid of it. For patients on PD, the usual target level for urea is below 25 mmol/l. For haemodialysis patients, the usual target levels are below 25 mmol/l before dialysis and below 9 mmol/l after dialysis.

Blood urea levels provide a less reliable guide than blood creatinine levels to your kidney, dialysis or transplant function. This is because the amount of urea in your blood is also affected by what you eat and by how much fluid there is in your body. If you eat a lot, or if you are dehydrated, the level of urea in your blood will rise.

4. Phosphate. The normal level of phosphate in your blood is 0.75–1.4 mmol/l. In normal quantities, phosphate helps calcium to strengthen the bones.

Healthy kidneys help to keep the right amount of phosphate in your blood. But if you have kidney failure, the level of phosphate in your blood will rise. (See *Chapter 6* for more information about phosphate and the bones.)

Phosphate is a dialysable substance, and the aim is to reduce the amount of phosphate in the blood of people with kidney failure. This is the reason that there is no phosphate in dialysis fluid. Phosphate therefore passes from the patient's blood into the dialysis fluid (because of the basic principle of dialysis, by which substances pass from a stronger to a weaker solution).

The target phosphate level for dialysis patients is less than 1.8 mmol/l. It is not usually possible to achieve normal phosphate levels in dialysis patients. Dialysis is simply not good enough at removing phosphate from the blood. If dialysis does not keep blood phosphate at the target level, it may be necessary to take calcium carbonate tablets (as Calcichew, for example). Not only do these tablets give you calcium, they also reduce the level of phosphate in your blood by binding it together so that it can be passed out in faeces when you go to the toilet.

5. Bicarbonate. The normal level of bicarbonate in the blood is 22–29 mmol/l. If your blood bicarbonate is lower than this, it means there is too much acid in your blood. Acid is a waste product of food; like other wastes in the blood, it is normally removed by the kidneys. But if you have kidney failure, the level of acid in your blood goes up and the level of bicarbonate (the body's natural alkali) falls. If the levels of acid in your blood are not corrected sufficiently well over a period of time, this may contribute to malnutrition (loss of flesh weight, see *Chapter 14, page 105* for more information). Malnutrition is a common problem in dialysis patients.

The target level for bicarbonate is normal, preferably high-normal, say 26 mmol/l or over. For haemodialysis patients, this target applies after dialysis. It does not matter if the bicarbonate is always just above normal. It may even be a good thing for your nutrition.

In order to keep the acidity of the blood normal, dialysis fluid contains an alkali (a substance that is the opposite of an acid). In haemodialysis fluid, the alkali is either bicarbonate (at a concentration of 35 mmol/l) or acetate (at a concentration of 40 mmol/l). In PD fluid, the alkali is either bicarbonate (at a concentration of 40 mmol/l) or lactate, at a concentration of either 35 or 40 mmol/l. Both acetate and lactate are changed into bicarbonate inside the body.

The level of alkali in the dialysis fluid is higher than the level of alkali in the blood. Because alkali is dialysable, and because of the basic principle of dialysis, alkali passes from the dialysis fluid into the patient. In the blood, the alkali neutralises the acid and produces normal blood bicarbonate levels.

6. Calcium. Calcium is a mineral that strengthens the bones. One of the functions of the kidneys is to help to keep calcium in the bones. But if you have kidney failure, calcium will pass out of your bones. There is also a fall in the level of calcium in your blood. (See *Chapter 6* for more information about calcium and the bones.)

The normal level of calcium in the blood is 2.1–2.6 mmol/l. Calcium is a dialysable substance, which means that it can be given to kidney patients in the dialysis fluid.

If there is a higher concentration of calcium in the dialysis fluid than in the blood, calcium will pass into the blood during dialysis.

The level of calcium in dialysis fluid ranges from 2.0 to 3.5 mmol/l. Different doctors prefer different levels of calcium in the dialysis fluid – all have their advantages. Most dialysis fluids allow calcium to flow into the blood.

The target level for calcium is 2.4–2.5 mmol/l. This level, in the high-middle of the normal range, has been found to be better for kidney patients than a calcium level in the middle of the range.

If the dialysis fluid does not give you enough calcium to achieve the target level, it may be necessary for you to take calcium tablets (such as Calcichew, for example) or vitamin D tablets (usually as alfacalcidol) to help your body absorb calcium.

7. Sodium. Sodium is one of the minerals normally present in the blood. Its name is sometimes written as Na (pronounced 'N…a'), which is the chemical symbol for sodium. The normal level of sodium in the blood is 135–143 mmol/l. Sodium keeps water in the body, and helps to control the blood pressure. Some doctors think that keeping sodium levels low is important and recommend restricting the amount of salt you eat. In addition, we know that salty foods increase thirst, making it harder to limit the amount of fluid you drink.

Controlling the level of sodium in the blood is quite easy for people on dialysis. This is done by having a concentration of sodium in the dialysis fluid similar to that in the blood. (PD fluid contains 132 mmol/l of sodium; haemodialysis fluid contains 132–145 mmol/l.) Because the levels of sodium in the dialysis fluid and the blood are similar, dialysis does not have much effect on the blood sodium level and a normal level is usually achieved.

8. Glucose. The normal fasting level of glucose in the blood is 3.0–5.6 mmol/l. Glucose is a type of sugar, and it provides the body with energy. The amount of glucose in the blood is controlled by a substance called insulin, which is made in the pancreas (a gland in the upper abdomen). When someone has diabetes mellitus ('sugar diabetes'), either their pancreas does not make enough insulin, or their body is unable to use the insulin that is made. This means that their blood glucose level tends to be high.

Blood glucose levels are only usually a problem for those patients with kidney failure who also have diabetes. Blood glucose problems in these patients are due to the diabetes itself, rather than to the kidney failure that was caused by the diabetes.

For kidney patients who do not have diabetes, it is usually easy to achieve a normal blood glucose level. So blood glucose is not something that most dialysis patients have to worry about.

Although glucose is a dialysable substance, it does not do what people might expect it to do during dialysis. Firstly, for haemodialysis, the dialysis fluid contains an amount of glucose similar to that in the blood (about 5 mmol/l). As expected, given the basic principle of dialysis, very little glucose passes between the blood and the dialysis fluid.

Secondly, some of the dialysis fluid used for PD contains a lot of glucose. Even a weak bag will contain about 75.5 mmol/l (which is more than 10 times the normal blood level of glucose). In this case, it might be assumed that glucose would pour into the patient's body and cause problems, but in fact, the body deals with the glucose well because it enters the bloodstream slowly.

As the glucose enters the bloodstream, the pancreas produces insulin to bring the level of glucose in the blood back down to normal.

However, if a person has diabetes and can't use or make enough insulin, the blood glucose should keep going up. In fact it does not, usually. If a PD patient uses a lot of 'strong' bags (containing 3.86% glucose, compared with 1.36% in weak bags), the amount of glucose entering the blood may be too much for the pancreas to cope with. If a patient has diabetes, it may also upset diabetic control, making it necessary to inject more insulin, or to take more tablets. This extra glucose may make any patient (diabetic or not) put on body weight, usually as fat.

Given that glucose sometimes causes problems for PD patients, you may wonder if it is really necessary to include it in the dialysis fluid. In fact, the glucose in the PD fluid is there to perform one of the two major tasks of the kidney, i.e. to remove water from the body (ultrafiltration). Information about non-glucose solutions for PD is given in Chapter 9 (see *page 63*).

TESTS FOR NON-DIALYSABLE SUBSTANCES

The next group of blood tests to be looked at in this chapter are those which measure blood levels of various non-dialysable substances. Like the tests already described, these tests – measuring blood levels of albumin, and various substances such as bilirubin that show liver function – form part of the regular biochemistry test for patients with kidney failure.

Albumin. Albumin is a type of body protein. It is made in the liver and is present in the blood. The normal level of albumin in the blood is 34–48 g/l (grams per litre of blood).

The level of albumin in the blood is measured because of the information this provides about whether a patient is eating enough (especially enough protein). Kidney failure tends to reduce appetite. Also, during dialysis, some albumin and other proteins are lost into the dialysis fluid. Many kidney patients have a lower than normal blood albumin level. If a patient's blood albumin level is always low, malnutrition (loss of flesh weight, see *Chapter 14, page 105*) may have become a problem.

Unfortunately, the information obtained by measuring the blood albumin level is not very reliable. One difficulty is that the blood albumin decreases very quickly whenever a person is ill. This means that it is not possible to tell whether or not the malnutrition diagnosed by the test is really a long-term problem. Another problem with the test is that the blood albumin tends to fall whatever is wrong with a patient, no matter how well nourished they are. So, for example, if you have any infection anywhere in your body, your blood albumin level will fall. A further problem with this test is that, even if a fall in the blood albumin level is identified, there are no specific treatments to bring it back up again. The target level, for what it is worth, is normal.

LIVER FUNCTION TESTS

The results of a group of tests called liver function tests (LFTs) often appear at the bottom of biochemistry test results. Most doctors do not mention these, or brush over them, saying 'Oh, don't worry about them, they are just liver tests'. So why are they measured? The main reason is that biochemistry tests are generally done by a machine, which includes the liver tests automatically.

Having said that, patients with kidney failure can get liver problems. Haemodialysis, blood transfusions or a kidney transplant puts patients at increased risk of catching a viral infection (such as hepatitis B or hepatitis C) that can cause liver failure. Also, some of the drugs used to suppress the immune system after a kidney transplant can affect the liver. This is particularly true for azathioprine, ciclosporin and tacrolimus.

So here is a quick guide to common LFTs:

1. Bilirubin. This is the most important of the LFTs. (It is the liver function equivalent of the creatinine test.) Bilirubin is produced when worn-out red blood cells are broken down for removal from the body. The normal range of level for bilirubin in the blood is 4–25 mmol/l. Raised bilirubin levels show that the liver is not working properly. If the blood bilirubin goes above 50 μmol/l, the patient will develop jaundice (go yellow in colour).

2. Alanine transaminase. The normal range for alanine transaminase (ALT) in the blood is 5–50 iu/l (international units per litre). Raised levels indicate that the liver cells have been damaged by disease.

3. Alkaline phosphatase. The normal range for alkaline phosphatase (alk. phos.) in the blood is 30–120 iu/l. This test measures how well bile (a liquid made by the liver) drains from the liver. Bile contains the waste products from the liver. It is drained into the bowel, and leaves the body in the faeces. In patients with kidney failure, a high alk. phos. level can also indicate renal bone disease as alk. phos. is involved in the bones, as well as the liver.

4. Gamma-glutamyltransferase. The normal range for gamma-glutamyltransferase (gammaGT) in the blood is 5–70 iu/l. Like alkaline phosphatase measurements, this test measures how well bile drains from the liver. GammaGT also rises if a patient drinks alcohol heavily over a number of years. A raised level can be an early sign of cirrhosis.

OTHER BLOOD TESTS

Kidney patients are also given a number of other blood tests in addition to the tests that make up their usual biochemistry test. The substances measured by these tests – haemoglobin (Hb), ferritin, cholesterol and parathyroid hormone – are all non-dialysable. Kidney patients have their Hb level measured each time they have a biochemistry blood test. Their blood levels of ferritin, cholesterol and parathyroid hormone are measured less often, usually every 3 months or so.

1. Haemoglobin. Most patients with some kidney failure have anaemia. Anaemia means that there is not enough of a substance called haemoglobin in the blood. Haemoglobin is important because it carries oxygen around the body. Every part of the body needs a regular supply of oxygen. (See *Chapter 5* for more information about anaemia in kidney patients.) The normal level of Hb is 11–17 g/dl (grams per decilitre of blood). If the Hb level is below 11.0 g/dl, the patient is said to be anaemic.

There is a very good treatment for anaemia called an erythropoietin stimulating agent (ESA), which is given as an injection between three times per week, and once every two weeks. Dialysis patients who are not being treated with an ESA may have an Hb of only 6–8 g/dl, which is very low. The aim of ESA treatment is to increase the Hb level to 11–12 g/dl. (See *Chapter 5* for more information on anaemia and its treatment.)

2. Ferritin. You need to have enough iron in your body if ESAs (see *above*) are to work well. The best guide to how much iron there is in the body is a blood test that measures the level of a substance called ferritin. The more iron there is in the body, the higher the level of ferritin in the blood and, generally speaking, the higher the levels the better.

For an ESA to work, it is important to have a ferritin level of at least 200 µg/l (micrograms per litre of blood). The normal level of ferritin is 15–350 µg/l, but 200 µg/l is generally considered an adequate level.

To keep the ferritin above 200 µg/l, many patients on ESAs need to take iron tablets, or have regular iron injections. Some renal units now give iron injections to all patients with kidney failure, whether or not they are on ESAs.

3. Cholesterol. Cholesterol is a form of fat present in the blood. High levels are thought to put people at risk of heart attacks and strokes. Current recommendations are to keep the level below 5 mmol/l of blood.

If the level of cholesterol in the blood is high, it can be reduced in some patients by going on a low-fat diet. However, many patients also need to take a tablet called a statin to control the levels.

4. Parathyroid hormone. Parathyroid hormone (PTH) is a hormone (a chemical messenger) that is made by four glands in the front of the neck. These glands are too small for you to see or feel them. If someone with kidney failure has low levels of calcium and/or high levels of phosphate for a long time, these glands grow and start producing too much PTH.

It is important to measure the level of PTH in the blood of people with kidney failure because of the information this test can provide about the bones. The amount of PTH in the blood is the best long-term guide to how much damage kidney failure has done to the bones. Blood levels of calcium and phosphate tell you

what is happening now; PTH also tells you what will happen in the future and, generally speaking, the higher the levels, the worse the bones.

Different renal units use different tests for measuring PTH, and different doctors have different views about PTH targets for kidney patients. The normal range is 1.1–4.2 pmol/l. Most doctors agree that a PTH level that is less than twice the upper limit of normal (i.e. less than 10 pmol/l) is generally considered to be satisfactory. As with phosphate levels, it is often hard to achieve normal PTH levels in people who have kidney failure. (See *Chapter 6* for more information about PTH and renal bone disease.)

OTHER TESTS

There are a number of other tests that patients are likely to experience at some time in the course of their life with kidney failure. The more common tests are described below. Some of these tests involve risks. You should always ask your doctor how a particular test will change your treatment and what the risks are before you agree to it. Not all tests that carry risk require a consent form (a CT scan doesn't, for example). So you can't even say, 'No consent form, no risk'.

For more information about tests while preparing for a transplant, see *Chapter 11, pages 82–3.*

FINDING OUT ABOUT KIDNEY FAILURE

1. Kidney biopsy. This test involves a hollow needle being used to remove a very small piece of the kidney, which can then be studied under a microscope. Biopsies are sometimes used to find out the cause of kidney failure. They are also used to check whether a transplanted kidney is being rejected.

If you are having a biopsy, you will be given a local anaesthetic to numb the area where the needle will be inserted. If a biopsy is being taken of your own

SUMMARY OF NORMAL AND TARGET BLOOD TEST RESULTS FOR PATIENTS ON DIALYSIS

Substance	Relevance	Normal level	Target level	Units
Dialysable substances				
Potassium	Heart health	3.7–5.0	normal	mmol/l
Creatinine	Toxin clearance	50–120	less than 600	µmol/l
Urea	Toxin clearance	2.6–6.6	less than 25	mmol/l
Phosphate	Bone health	0.75–1.4	less than 1.8	mmol/l
Bicarbonate	Acid balance	22–29	high–normal (26–29)	mmol/l
Calcium	Bone health	2.1–2.6	high–normal (2.4–2.5)	mmol/l
Sodium	Fluid balance	135–143	normal	mmol/l
Glucose (fasting)	Blood sugar	3.0–5.6	normal	mmol/l
Non-dialysable substances				
Albumin	Nutritional status	34–48	normal	g/l
Bilirubin	Liver function	4–25	normal	mmol/l
ALT	Liver function	5–50	normal	iu/l
Alk. phos.	Liver function	30–120	normal	iu/l
GammaGT	Liver function	5–70	normal	iu/l
Other (non-dialysable) substances				
Haemoglobin	Blood health	11–17	11–12	g/dl
Ferritin	Iron in blood	15–350	more than 200	µg/l
Cholesterol	Heart and brain health	3–6.0	less than 5	mmol/l
Parathyroid hormone	Bone health	1.1–4.2	less than 10	pmol/l

How do your test results compare? Although your hospital may use slightly different figures, they should be similar to those given here. If any of your figures do not seem to be on target, find out why.

kidneys, you will be asked to lie on your front. If the biopsy is being taken from a transplant kidney, you will need to lie on your back because a kidney transplant is placed in the front of the body, just above the groin. After a transplant, several biopsies may be necessary over the first few weeks. After the biopsy, you will need to rest for 6–12 hours, but it is usually possible to go home the next day (or even later the same day in some units).

Kidney biopsies have risks. There is a 1 in 20 chance that not enough kidney tissue will have been taken, meaning that the procedure will need to be repeated. There is also a 1 in 20 chance of seeing blood in the urine after the biopsy. This usually clears up on its own but, in 1 case in 100, a blood transfusion is required. Occasionally, the bleeding is so severe that the kidney has to be removed in an operation. If you already have kidney failure, this can lead to the need for dialysis which can be permanent. There is also a 1 in 1000 chance of a biopsy causing death. So biopsies should only be carried out if there is a good chance they will provide the doctors with information that will change your treatment. Always ask the doctor how the biopsy will affect your treatment before you agree to have one.

2. X-rays. Various types of X-ray are used to investigate kidney problems. X-rays may be taken of the kidneys, of the bladder – an **intravenous pyelogram (IVP)**, **intravenous urogram (IVU)** or **micturating cystourethrogram** – or of the blood vessels to the kidneys (**renal angiogram**, see *below*). These special X-ray tests usually require the use of radio-opaque dye (fluid which shows up on X-ray film), which may be injected into the bloodstream or flushed into the bladder during a cystoscopy (when a telescope is put into the bladder). There is also a small risk of worsening kidney function (as with renal angiograms), or even of causing death, with all of these tests as the dye is toxic to the kidneys. Always ask the doctor what effect it will have on your treatment before you agree to have one.

3. Renal angiogram. For this test, a special tube is passed into the femoral artery (a blood vessel in the groin). This plastic tube is fed up the artery, towards the kidney, and a special dye that shows up on X-rays is injected into it. The dye makes it possible to take X-ray pictures of the blood vessels of the kidney, which will show the doctors if there is anything blocking them.

A renal angiogram is a complex test which has risks. Possible side effects include bruising in the groin (common) and pain. The X-ray dye can be toxic to the kidneys and may damage them. There is a 5–15% risk that a renal angiogram will make the kidney function worse. Although this is quite high, the kidneys normally recover. There is a 2% chance of the dye causing so much damage that the person will need dialysis earlier than expected, though in many cases the kidneys will recover. A few patients will need dialysis permanently however. In addition, a small number of people may be allergic to the dye. Complications following an angiogram can cause death in around 1 in 1,000 cases. So (as for the renal biopsy) you should ask your doctor how the angiogram will change your treatment before you agree to have one.

4. Computed tomography (CT) scan. This is another special type of X-ray. It uses a machine to send X-rays around the area being looked at, in order to build up an image of the 'slice' of body being scanned. If you are having a CT scan, you will need to lie inside the machine for it to take place. You may also need to be injected with radio-opaque dye, and if you do – as with renal angiograms – there is a small risk it will make your kidney function worse. In very rare cases, the radio-opaque dye can even cause death.

5. Nuclear medicine scan. There are several types of nuclear medicine scan, which are becoming more popular as they are less likely to cause complications than X-rays, angiograms or CT scans. All nuclear medicine scans involve the injection of a small amount of a radio-active substance into the bloodstream. An 'isotope GFR' (glomerular filtration rate) is the most accurate way of measuring the kidney function – even more accurate than measuring creatinine level, eGFR or creatinine clearance. A 'DMSA scan' looks at the structure of the kidney (and is good for diagnosing reflux nephropathy, see *page* 6). A 'DTPA scan' is used for comparing the function of each kidney, i.e. to find out which one is working harder. (They should work equally hard.) A 'MAG-3 scan' is good at looking at both structure and function. The risks involved with having nuclear medicine scans are low.

6. MRI scan. MRI stands for magnetic resonance imaging – a scanning technique which uses magnetism, radio waves and a computer to produce high-quality pictures of the inside of the body. For an MRI scan, you will need to lie inside a large machine that sends signals to a computer. The computer then builds an image of the inside of your body. No X-rays are used. An MRI scan allows doctors to see good pictures of the inside of the kidney, which will help them to discover what is causing your problems. It often produces better quality pictures than a CT scan.

7. Ultrasound scans. This is the same type of test as that used on pregnant women to check on the baby in the womb. It is also used to help discover the cause of kidney problems – either when kidney failure is first discovered, or if there appear to be problems after a transplant. It uses sound waves, so is completely safe.

Jelly is spread on the skin and an ultrasound probe moved over the abdomen and sides of the body, allowing the kidneys to be seen on the screen. Sometimes, the person carrying out the test may print photographs of certain images seen on the screen. The test is quick and painless for the patient, and tells the doctor if a kidney is shrunken, enlarged or even missing.

Ultrasound scans may be used to allow the doctor to locate the kidney before taking a biopsy.

TESTS FOR PEOPLE ON DIALYSIS

1. Adequacy test. Adequacy is a general term that refers to how well dialysis is working. Adequacy tests are basically **clearance tests**, as described in *Chapter 2, pages 16–17*.

2. Peritoneal equilibration test (PET). This is a test for patients who are being treated by peritoneal dialysis (see *Chapter 9*). The test measures how quickly waste products and fluid are removed from the blood during dialysis. It is an important test in determining the correct prescription for peritoneal dialysis. The test takes place over 4 hours, and involves taking samples of dialysis fluid and a blood test at 2 hourly intervals. Other similar tests include the **peritoneal function test (PFT)** when samples are taken from all the used dialysis fluid.

3. Residual renal function (RRF). When patients first start dialysis, their own kidneys may still be working, but at a reduced level. The amount they are still working will vary from patient to patient and is known as 'residual renal function'. The longer a patient keeps their RRF, the healthier they will be. Over time, it is likely the RRF will decline, and in many patients, it eventually disappears altogether. As the RRF declines, the dialysis prescription should be adjusted to make up for the reduced function. A **creatinine clearance test**, which measures the amount of creatinine cleared by the kidneys and put into the urine (see *Chapter 2, pages 16–17*), is used to assess RRF.

KEY FACTS

1 The term 'figures' is used to refer to the biochemistry blood test that most kidney patients have at the end of every clinic appointment.

2 The biochemistry test is not a single blood test. It measures the levels of a dozen or so different substances in the blood. The results tell you and your doctor about the levels of minerals in your body, the acidity of your blood, and the state of your bones. It will also give information about how well nourished you are, and how well your kidneys are working.

3 The substances that are measured can be divided into two groups: dialysable and non-dialysable.

4 Dialysable substances can pass from the blood into the dialysis fluid and vice versa. Substances pass from a stronger to a weaker solution. This basic principle of dialysis determines the direction in which a substance travels during dialysis.

5 Potassium, creatinine, urea and phosphate are dialysable substances that are taken out of the body during dialysis.

6 Calcium and bicarbonate are dialysable substances that are usually put into the body during dialysis.

7 Non-dialysable substances measured by blood tests include albumin, various substances that measure liver function, haemoglobin, ferritin, cholesterol and parathyroid hormone.

8 If you have kidney failure, you should know the values of most of your blood tests. Ask for the results after each blood test is done.

9 If you have kidney failure, you may need other tests to find out about the extent to which your kidneys have failed, tests to see how well dialysis is working for you, and tests to prepare you for a transplant.

10 Tests for finding out about kidney failure and dialysis include biopsies and angiograms, clearance tests and various types of imaging and X-ray. Ask about the risks of these tests before you agree to have one.

8 DIALYSIS – THE BASICS

This chapter describes what dialysis is, and explains how it works. It also discusses the consequences of having dialysis at home or in the renal unit.

INTRODUCTION

This is the first of six chapters which explain the treatment options available to people with kidney failure. There are basically two ways of treating kidney failure: dialysis (see also *Chapters 9 and 10*) and transplantation (see *Chapters 11, 12 and 13*). There is currently no cure. In other words, dialysis and/or a kidney transplant can replace some of the function of two kidneys (a transplant at most 60%; dialysis 5%) but does not get rid of the underlying problem. Kidney doctors will still consider that you have kidney failure, whether you are pre-dialysis, on dialysis or have a kidney transplant.

WHAT IS DIALYSIS?

Dialysis is an artificial way of doing the work of the kidneys. It clears waste products from the blood, and it also removes excess water. The word 'dialysis' comes from a Greek word meaning 'to separate' – because dialysis separates the waste and water from the blood, and removes them from the body. It therefore performs the two main functions of the kidneys: toxin clearance (see *Chapter 2*) and maintaining fluid balance (see *Chapter 3*).

There are two different types of dialysis: peritoneal dialysis (see *Chapter 9*), and haemodialysis (see *Chapter 10*).

DIALYSIS AT HOME OR IN THE RENAL UNIT?

Almost everyone who has kidney failure will need to have dialysis during their lifetime. It's therefore important to consider **where** you would prefer to have your treatment; at home or in hospital, when making a decision about the type of dialysis. Both forms of dialysis are equally effective and most people are suitable for either PD or haemodialysis. Most patients will experience both PD and haemodialysis at different times.

PD is a done in a home setting whereas haemodialysis can be done either at home or in a dialysis unit.

When choosing where to have dialysis, the following points should be taken into consideration:

- **Flexibility of treatment.** Having dialysis in the renal unit usually means that patients have fixed treatment appointments three times a week for four hours each. This enables patients to have four days 'off' dialysis every week. Dialysis at home is more flexible, but it is usually done every day. Both PD and home haemodialysis can be done overnight, leaving day times free for work, study or family commitments. Renal unit-based haemodialysis is not very flexible. But in some units it can be done overnight.

- **Work.** Many dialysis patients are able to continue to work. Fixed dialysis schedules can be altered to accommodate work patterns; however those on home-based dialysis usually find it easier to continue their employment. The nurses at the dialysis unit will be happy to speak to a patient's employer about working while on dialysis.

- **Travel to the dialysis unit.** People who have dialysis 'in-centre' (i.e. at the main hospital renal unit) will need to make arrangements to get to the unit three times a week. It may be possible for transport to be provided by the hospital, or you might be able to make your own way there. Whatever method of transport is chosen, the time taken to travel to and from the dialysis centre should be taken into consideration. Hospital transport is not reliable in some units. This can turn the four hours of dialysis into eight hours of frustration, waiting for transport.

- **Space for supplies and treatment.** Dialysis at home requires space to store supplies. Most home dialysis patients will need to store at least one month's supplies. The equipment can be stored in the garage, a shed, in the cupboard under the stairs or a spare room. Space also needs to be set aside for the dialysis to be performed. This may need to be in the bedroom if night-time dialysis is chosen.

- **Holidays and travel.** It is possible to have dialysis away from home. PD patients can have their supplies delivered to their destination. And although this requires forward planning, travel for holidays, family events or business can usually be arranged to most parts of the world. More planning is usually required for haemodialysis patients as they need to find a centre in which they can have their treatment while they are away from home. The renal unit will help with the arrangements for both haemodialysis and PD patients to have dialysis away from home.

- **Contact with other patients.** People who have haemodialysis in the main hospital or satellite unit, have regular contact with other patients each time they attend for treatment. People on home-based treatments will meet patients if they attend clinics, patient groups or are admitted to hospital.

- **Contact with healthcare professionals.** Having haemodialysis in the main hospital or satellite unit means that there is a healthcare professional present during each dialysis session. People who have dialysis at home will have regular contact with healthcare professionals through home visits, telephone contact and regular clinic visits. Anyone who has home dialysis will be trained and educated about all aspects of their treatment. Some people who have dialysis at home can have daily assistance from a carer. This might be a paid carer, a relative or partner.

In the UK about 21% of dialysis patients are currently treated at home, whereas in the late 1980s about 50% of dialysis patients had their treatment at home. There are a number of possible reasons for this decline. In the 1990s, investment in dialysis provision from the government led to the building of many new haemodialysis 'satellite' units. These centres were built closer to patients' homes making hospital-like dialysis more convenient for some people. In addition, the increasing age of the population means that many older people now start dialysis. Some doctors do not think that home-based treatments are suitable for older people; however there is no evidence to support this view.

The situation is now beginning to change. There are

many government initiatives calling for people to have the opportunity to receive treatment for a chronic illness at home. Help is now available for people to be supported to have home dialysis. In addition, new technologies are being developed that will make home dialysis even more convenient and flexible for patients and their families.

HOW DOES DIALYSIS WORK?

PD and haemodialysis work in similar ways:

- Waste products are cleared from the blood by a process called diffusion (see *page 54*).

- Excess water is removed from the blood by a process known as ultrafiltration (see *page 54*).

- Wastes and water pass into a special liquid – called the dialysis fluid or dialysate – for removal from the body.

- A thin layer of tissue or plastic, known as the dialysis membrane, keeps the dialysis fluid and blood apart.

In PD, the dialysis takes place all the time as the dialysis fluid is always in contact with the dialysis membrane. Haemodialysis is usually done intermittently; either four hours, up to three times a week for renal unit-based haemodialysis, or more frequently (either daily for fewer hours, or overnight) for home haemodialysis.

PD and haemodialysis are equivalent techniques in terms of the amount of dialysis they can deliver (about 5% of the function of two normal kidneys) which is sufficient to relieve the symptoms of kidney failure.

THE ROLE OF THE DIALYSIS FLUID

Both of the key processes involved in dialysis – i.e.

diffusion and ultrafiltration – depend on the use of a dialysis fluid. Body wastes and excess fluid can only pass from the blood if they have somewhere to go. The dialysis fluid provides the 'container' in which they are removed from the body. The dialysis solution is slightly different in each type of dialysis, but it does the same job.

The chemical content of the dialysis fluid affects the flow of substances between the blood and the dialysis fluid. During dialysis, body wastes and excess fluid pass from the blood into the dialysis fluid. Other substances, usually 'good' ones such as calcium, flow in the opposite direction, from the dialysis fluid into the blood.

THE DIALYSIS MEMBRANE

Dialysis solution is toxic to the body if it flows directly into the blood. It is important therefore to keep the dialysis fluid separate from the blood. This is done by using a dialysis membrane, which looks similar to a very thin piece of 'cling film'.

The dialysis membrane has thousands of tiny holes in it. These holes are big enough to let water, body wastes and various other substances through, yet small enough to keep the blood cells and proteins inside the blood vessels. So the dialysis membrane acts as a 'leaky barrier' between the blood and the dialysis fluid.

In haemodialysis, the membrane used is artificial, made from a type of plastic. The membrane, folded over many thousands of times, is situated in an artificial kidney (called a dialyser). Dialysis takes place outside the patient's body, in the artificial kidney.

In PD, a natural membrane inside the abdomen, called the peritoneum, is used. The peritoneum lines the inside wall of the abdomen, and covers all the abdominal organs (the stomach, bowels, liver, etc.). It is a thin layer of tissue, rather like a thin balloon in appearance and texture.

WASTE REMOVAL BY DIFFUSION

Diffusion is one of the key processes involved in dialysis. It is a process by which substances pass from a stronger to a weaker solution.

Diffusion works in the same way as a tea bag. When hot water is poured over a tea bag, the tea comes out of the bag and into the water. The surface of the tea bag is like the dialysis membrane, as it lets tea drain out of the tea leaves, but does not let the tea leaves out themselves. The tea mixes with the water until the tea is the same colour throughout the cup.

People with kidney failure have a lot of body wastes in their blood. If the blood is put next to a dialysis fluid that does not have any of these wastes in it, the wastes will pass from the blood into the dialysis fluid. So, if we want to remove unwanted substances (such as urea or creatinine) from the blood, we need a dialysis fluid that contains little or none of those substances.

As dialysis proceeds, there comes a point at which there are equal amount of wastes in the blood and in the dialysis fluid (as when the tea stops changing colour). The process of diffusion then stops, and no more wastes will move across. This is the basic principle underlying dialysis.

Diffusion also works the 'other way' round. If the amount of a substance is higher in the dialysis fluid than in the blood, then that substance will pass from the dialysis fluid into the blood. So if we want to add useful substances (such as calcium and bicarbonate) to the body via the blood, we use dialysis fluid that contains a lot of those substances.

FLUID REMOVAL BY ULTRAFILTRATION

Ultrafiltration – the other key process involved in dialysis – occurs at the same time as diffusion. It is the process by which excess fluid (mainly water) is drawn out of the blood during dialysis. Ultrafiltration

The process of diffusion

1

2

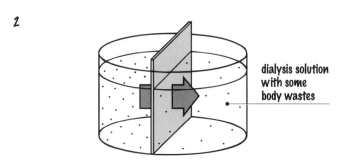

Blood cells are too big to pass through the dialysis membrane, but body wastes begin to diffuse (pass) into the dialysis solution

3

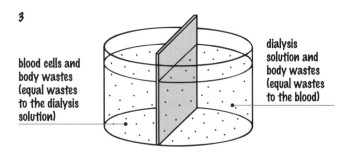

Diffusion is complete. Body wastes have diffused through the membrane, and now there are equal amounts of wastes in both the blood and the dialysis solution

happens in slightly different ways in haemodialysis and PD.

In haemodialysis, the water is 'sucked' from the blood by the kidney machine using negative pressure. The amount of water to be removed during a session of haemodialysis can be varied, from a lot to a little, depending on how the machine is set up.

In PD, a substance is put into the dialysis fluid which 'sucks' the water from the blood. The most commonly used substance is glucose (i.e. sugar). The way the glucose sucks water from the blood is the same way as a tree draws water up from the ground to its highest leaves. It depends on a process called osmosis.

Osmosis occurs when a liquid from a weak solution (e.g. water in the blood) passes through a semi-permeable membrane (e.g. the dialysis membrane) into a stronger solution (e.g. one of glucose in the dialysis fluid). By this means, water is lost from the blood, and the glucose solution is diluted.

The amount of water drawn from the blood depends on the amount of sugar in the solution – the more sugar, the more water will be removed. Hence in PD, there are different strengths of dialysis bag – with 'strong' bags containing more sugar than 'weak' bags. The choice of bag depends on how much water needs to be removed from the patient's blood: a strong bag will remove more water than a weak bag.

The process of ultrafiltration in PD

1

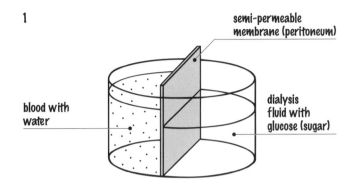

blood with water

semi-permeable membrane (peritoneum)

dialysis fluid with glucose (sugar)

2

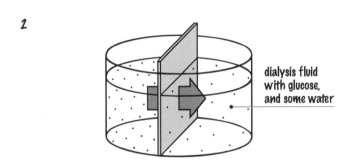

dialysis fluid with glucose, and some water

Blood cells are too big to pass through the semi-permeable membrane, but water in the blood is drawn into the dialysis fluid by the glucose

3

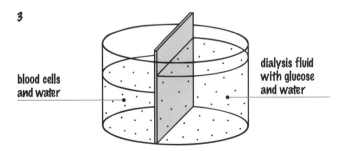

blood cells and water

dialysis fluid with glucose and water

Ultrafiltration is complete. Water has been drawn through the peritoneum by the glucose in the dialysis fluid. There is now extra water in the dialysis fluid, which needs to be changed

KEY FACTS

1 Dialysis is the word used to describe the removal of body wastes and water from the blood.

2 There are two types of dialysis: haemodialysis and peritoneal dialysis (PD). Both work in a similar way.

3 PD is done in the home setting whereas haemodialysis can be done at home or in a hospital or satellite (local) unit.

4 Most patients can have either type of dialysis, and may well experience both at different times.

5 There are two main processes involved in dialysis: diffusion and ultrafiltration. Diffusion removes the body wastes, and ultrafiltration removes the excess water.

9 PERITONEAL DIALYSIS

This chapter concentrates on peritoneal dialysis (PD), a form of dialysis that is used to treat people with kidney failure at home.

INTRODUCTION

Peritoneal dialysis (PD) is a form of dialysis used to treat people with kidney failure at home. In PD, the process of dialysis (see *Chapter 8*) takes place inside the patient's body, using the peritoneum (the natural lining of the abdomen) as the dialysis membrane. PD has been available in the UK since the late 1970s and is the most widely used form of home dialysis.

HOW DOES PD WORK?

PD is a continuous treatment that takes over some of the work which is normally done by the kidneys. It removes the waste products of food (toxin clearance, see *Chapter 2*), and removes excess water from the body (see *Chapter 3*).

The basic principles of dialysis are the same for PD and haemodialysis. (These principles are explained in detail in *Chapter 8*.) Briefly, dialysis uses a special liquid (called the dialysis fluid, dialysis solution or dialysate) and a membrane (called the dialysis membrane) which acts as a filter. In PD, the dialysis membrane is the patient's own peritoneum (see *below*).

The dialysis fluid provides the 'container' into which waste products and excess water can be removed from the body. The dialysis membrane keeps the dialysis fluid and the blood separate from each other, and is the filter that allows certain substances and water to pass through it. Substances pass from the blood into the dialysis fluid (and vice versa). They do this by a process called diffusion, by which substances pass from a stronger to a weaker solution (see *page 54*).

At the same time, ultrafiltration occurs (see *page 54*). Excess water passes from the blood into the dialysis fluid by a process called osmosis, in which liquid in a weaker solution passes into a stronger one. In PD, the dialysis happens continuously because there is always dialysis fluid in contact with the peritoneal membrane.

PD is a home-based therapy that patients usually do themselves. It is a flexible treatment that can be carried out anywhere there is a convenient place. Although the vast majority of patients do PD for themselves, some patients have help from a carer to do some or all of their dialysis. This is called assisted PD.

THE PERITONEUM

In PD, the dialysis process takes place continuouously inside the patient's abdomen, using a natural membrane – the peritoneum – as the dialysis membrane. It is from the peritoneum that PD (peritoneal dialysis) gets its name.

The peritoneum is a natural membrane that lines the inside of the abdominal wall and covers all the abdominal organs (the stomach, bowels, liver, etc.). It resembles a balloon in appearance and texture but has lots of extremely tiny holes in it. These holes allow the peritoneum to be used as a dialysis membrane. As blood flows through the blood vessels in the peritoneum, it flows past the holes. Although the holes are extremely tiny, water and toxins can easily pass through, but blood cells are too large. In this way, the peritoneum in PD works as a 'natural filter'.

The peritoneum has two layers – one lining the inside of the abdominal wall, the other lining the abdominal organs. Between these two layers is a space. This space is called the peritoneal cavity. Normally, the peritoneal cavity contains only about 100 ml of liquid. During PD, it is the peritoneal cavity that is used as a reservoir for the dialysis fluid. In fact, it can expand to hold a few litres of fluid.

How is PD done?

PD is a continuous therapy meaning that the levels of waste products and fluid in the body do not rise and fall as much as they do with unit-based haemodialysis, which is usually done three times a week. Dialysis takes place all the time as the fluid is constantly in contact with the peritoneal membrane. The process consists of the following three stages:

1. The peritoneal cavity is filled with 1.5–3 litres of dialysis fluid from a dialysis bag. (The amount varies, depending on a patient's individual needs and the type of dialysis fluid used.) The fluid drains into the peritoneal cavity by gravity.

2. The dialysis fluid is left inside the peritoneum to allow dialysis to take place. (The length of time it stays there

The position of the peritoneal cavity

varies, from between 1 and 8 hours, depending on individual requirements, the time of day and the type of PD.)

3. The 'used' fluid, containing the water and waste products that the kidneys would normally have passed into the urine, is drained out of the body by gravity and is thrown away, usually down the toilet.

OPERATION TO INSERT A PD CATHETER

The dialysis fluid gets in and out of the peritoneal cavity via a small plastic tube that is placed into the abdomen. The tube is inserted during a short operation (which is performed using either a local or a general anaesthetic), and will remain in place permanently, until PD is no longer required (see *diagram*). This tube is called a PD catheter. It is about 30 centimetres (12 inches) long and as wide as a pencil.

The PD catheter will be placed through your lower abdominal wall, into your peritoneal cavity. Half of the catheter lies inside your abdomen, and half lies outside. It will come out on the right or the left usually under your navel (tummy button). The PD catheter acts as a permanent pathway into your peritoneal cavity from the outside world. Without it, you won't be able to perform PD, so it is important you look after it.

The operation to insert the catheter can be done as a

PD catheter – position inside the body

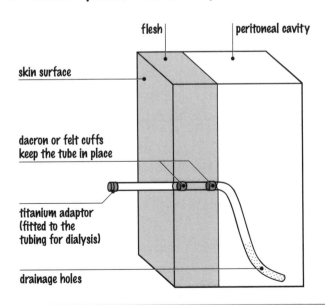

flesh

peritoneal cavity

skin surface

dacron or felt cuffs keep the tube in place

titanium adaptor (fitted to the tubing for dialysis)

drainage holes

'day case' meaning that you won't need to stay in hospital overnight. The catheter is usually 'left alone' for 7–10 days or more after the operation. This allows it to 'settle in' and gives the abdominal wound time to heal. Occasionally, however, it may need to be used straight away if dialysis is needed urgently. Sometimes the PD catheter does not work first time and another short operation will be needed to resolve the problem. This might be a 'repositioning' or an 'omentectomy' (the removal of fat that has got in the way).

THE TRAINING

PD is a home-based treatment, usually done by patients themselves. It is important, therefore, that anyone having PD is properly trained. This training is usually given to patients, and a partner if preferred, two weeks after their PD catheter operation.

Patients are fully trained in all aspects of their care by specialist nurses. Most patients can become competent in the exchange technique in 3–14 days. Some hospitals train people as in-patients, others train them as out-patients, and some patients are trained at home. When patients first go home and have to do the exchanges by themselves, they may find it a bit daunting. However, within a few days or weeks most patients find they are doing dialysis by themselves with no problems. In some situations, individuals are able to have support from a specially trained healthcare worker to help with their dialysis. This may be a temporary measure, with the support worker visiting the person for the first few weeks while confidence is built up. Other people need the support for longer, and others have permanent support.

METHODS OF FLUID EXCHANGE

The way that the dialysis fluid is exchanged depends on the type of PD. There are two main types of PD, which differ only in the way that the dialysis fluid is exchanged. The two different types of PD are:

Fluid exchanges in CAPD

1

2

3

4

5

a peritoneal cavity
b catheter tube

1 Patient with used dialysis fluid ready to exchange

2 A Y-shaped tube is connected to the patient's PD catheter. At one end of the Y tubing is a bag full of fresh dialysis fluid (A). Used fluid is drained into the empty bag (B), which is at the other end of the Y tubing

3 When all the used fluid has drained into the drainage bag (B), the drainage tube is clamped to stop more fluid flowing down the tube. The seal is broken and fresh fluid is then drained into the peritoneal cavity from bag A

4 Once all the fresh fluid is inside the patient, all the tubes are clamped and the bags are disconnected, leaving the patient free from the equipment until the next time a dialysis exchange is due

5 Patient with fresh dialysis fluid

1. Continuous ambulatory peritoneal dialysis (CAPD). 'Continuous' means 'all the time' and 'ambulatory' means 'while you walk around'. In this form of PD, the dialysis solution is changed manually.

2. Automated peritoneal dialysis (APD). 'Automated' means that a machine changes the dialysis fluid for the patient. The patient remains connected to the machine while dialysis is taking place, at night while they are asleep (see *below*).

FLUID EXCHANGES IN CAPD

CAPD involves draining 1.5–3 litres of dialysis fluid into your abdomen, leaving it there for 4–8 hours, and then draining it out. This is done four or five times a day – every day. It is as simple as that. With practice, an exchange of fluid can be done in less than 30 minutes. Exchanges are simple to do and can be performed almost anywhere, and you can watch TV, read etc. while it is happening.

The dialysis fluid is kept in sealed plastic bags. The bags are connected and disconnected to the peritoneal catheter with a system of tubes and clamps. (How this is done is shown in the diagrams on *page 60*.) There are no 'set' times to carry out the exchanges. However, a 4-bag regime 'fits' into a typical day. For example, the first bag might be exchanged at breakfast, the second at lunchtime, the third before the evening meal, and the fourth before going to bed (leaving the fluid for the last exchange in through the night). It is easy for patients to adapt the timing of exchanges to their own individual needs. For example, if you want to go out for the day, you could delay your mid-day exchange, and do two 'quick bags' (say, three hours apart) after coming home. It may be safe to miss the occasional bag, but this is certainly not recommended on a regular basis. You should always check with your doctor or nurse before doing this.

FLUID EXCHANGES IN APD

APD uses a machine to do the dialysis fluid exchanges. Most people have their machine in the bedroom, where it does the exchanges while they are asleep. APD machines are quite compact, about the size of a small suitcase (*see above*) which makes it possible for patients to do exchanges anywhere there is an electricity supply.

Most patients need to spend 7–10 hours attached to the machine every night. This enables the machine to perform an average of six exchanges of 1.5–3 litres of dialysis fluid each night. The length of time that PD fluid is left in the abdomen before it is exchanged by the machine varies between about one and three hours. After spending the night on the machine, most people on APD keep fluid inside their peritoneum during the daytime without needing to exchange it.

A few patients can afford to miss one night's dialysis very occasionally. However, they should always check first with the doctor or nurse at the renal unit to see whether this is safe.

A portable APD machine

control panel | heater | dialysis bag | extra supply of dialysis bags

drain ◄ ——— ► patient

CAPD OR APD?

In most renal units in the UK, about 60% of the PD patients currently do CAPD, and 40% do APD. However, the number of patients doing APD is growing all the time. Different patients may be better suited to either CAPD or APD for a number of reasons:

1. Lifestyle choices. APD is done during the night which means that the daytime is left free for patients to carry on their normal activities. For this reason, APD is often chosen by people who work or have a family to care for. APD is also more appropriate for people who need assistance to perform some or all of their dialysis. The machine can be set up and/or dismantled by a carer, taking away some of the responsibility of dialysis.

2. How the peritoneum works. The main medical reason why a doctor may choose either CAPD or APD for a patient relates to the way the patient's peritoneum works during dialysis.

Some patients, have a peritoneal membrane which works best with more frequent exchanges of dialysis fluid. This type of membrane, called a 'high transport membrane' is usually more suited to APD, because the machine is able to do rapid exchanges of dialysis fluid while they sleep.

Other patients, called 'low transporters', will get more dialysis if the fluid is left inside them for longer periods. Low transporters are generally better suited to CAPD.

A test has been developed to find out whether patients are 'high' or 'low transporters'. This test is called a peritoneal equilibration test (see page 49), and is usually performed in hospital by a nurse. It takes place over four hours, and involves taking samples of PD fluid at 2-hourly intervals along with one blood sample. The test measures how quickly the waste products and excess water move out of the patient's bloodstream and into the dialysis fluid. If the waste products move quickly, the patient is called a 'high transporter'. If the waste products move slowly, the patient is a 'low transporter'.

3. Patient size. APD can also be particularly good for patients who require a lot of dialysis – for example, large people, especially those who no longer pass urine. This is because the machine can do more fluid exchanges (and therefore more dialysis), than patients are able to do themselves with CAPD. Also, as the patients are lying down, they may be more able to tolerate bigger volumes of dialysis fluid. (This is because there is less pressure on the abdomen when you are lying down.)

In these ways, APD can remove more waste products than CAPD. Even so, for some very large patients, APD during the night may not be enough. Such patients commonly need an additional CAPD exchange at tea-time.

DIFFERENT AMOUNTS AND TYPES OF PD FLUID

Whatever the type of PD (either CAPD or APD), the ability to remove toxins (i.e. clearance) can be raised by increasing either the volume of fluid used, or the number of exchanges, or both. A larger volume of dialysis fluid will remove more waste products (and a little more water) than a smaller volume of dialysis fluid. The dialysis needs of patients depend partly on their body size (see Chapter 2). Big people usually need more fluid (2.5 or 3 litres of dialysis fluid).

The ability of PD fluid to remove water (i.e. to do ultrafiltration) is affected by the amount of glucose (sugar) in the bag – the more glucose in the bag, the more water is removed. There are three different strengths: strong (3.86% glucose solution), medium (2.27% glucose) and weak (1.36% glucose). If you have too much water in your body (a condition called fluid overload, see page 21) you will be advised to use more strong or medium dialysis fluid. These will remove more water than weaker dialysis fluid.

The strength of the dialysis fluid is different from the volume, or amount of dialysis fluid used in each exchange. Strong fluid has more glucose in it than a weak fluid, but the amount used will be the same. Patients are advised to consider the weak (1.35%) fluid as their 'standard', and to try to use a minimum of stronger fluids. This is because it has been noticed that using a lot of high glucose fluid may damage the peritoneal membrane in the long term. This may mean that PD will not work effectively after many years of treatment.

ALTERNATIVE DIALYSIS FLUIDS

There are a number of other dialysis fluids available:

1. Icodextrin. This fluid contains a glucose polymer (in which the glucose molecules are very large), rather than ordinary glucose. Because the molecules are so large, they cannot pass through the peritoneal membrane. It is therefore good for those exchanges which take place over a longer period, either the day-time exchange for people on APD or the night-time one for people on CAPD. Icodextrin may also be recommended for PD patients who have diabetes or are overweight. This is because the glucose polymer in Icodextrin is less likely than ordinary glucose to be absorbed into the body to cause problems with sugar balance or weight gain. Icodextrin has also been shown to benefit patients who have been on PD for a long time and whose peritoneums do not work very well for dialysis.

2. Amino acids. Some other dialysis fluids use amino acids rather than glucose. This solution does not contain any glucose, which makes it particularly suitable for people with diabetes or people who are obese. As amino acids are the building blocks of protein, and as some of the amino acids are absorbed into the blood, it is thought that these dialysis fluids might also act as food supplements.

3. Bicarbonate. A bicarbonate-based dialysis fluid has been developed to help patients who have problems regulating the level of acid in their bodies. The solution is very similar to that of the human body (it is 'biocompatible'), and is thought to preserve the patient's peritoneal membrane. This solution may also be good for people who experience pain when the fluid is drained in. Bicarbonate solutions are rapidly becoming the most commonly used basic solutions, replacing lactate-based solutions.

WHO CAN BE TREATED BY PD?

PD is suitable for most people with established renal failure (ERF). There are only two reasons why PD might not be suitable. Either because the patient has a serious hernia that can't be surgically repaired. Or because the peritoneal membrane does not work. This might be due to adhesions (internal fibrous scars that form after an abdominal operation) or thickening of the peritoneal membrane. There is a condition called Encapsulating Peritoneal Sclerosis in which the peritoneal membrane can become thicker and stop working when a person has been on PD for a long time. Fortunately, this condition is extremely rare and happens in only 2% of people who have been on PD for longer than eight years.

LIVING WITH PD

Once people develop ERF, they will have it for the rest of their lives. Without treatment – by PD, haemo-dialysis or a kidney transplant – people with ERF will die within a few weeks. With treatment, they will be able to do all or most of the things they did before they became ill. PD does affect a person's lifestyle – especially because of the need for daily dialysis – but the limitations are often less of a problem than many people might expect.

1. Flexibility. PD is a flexible treatment which can be performed almost anywhere. The dialysis supplies can be delivered to most parts of the world, and APD machines are portable.

2. Independence. People on PD usually do their own dialysis, in their own homes. This gives many PD patients a greater sense of responsibility and independence than is possible for the majority of haemodialysis patients (who receive their dialysis from nurses or dialysis technicians in a hospital).

3. Sport and exercise. Most types of sport and exercise are possible for people on PD. Even contact sports are possible (although not always recommended).

4. Swimming/baths/showers. It's possible for PD patients to go swimming. Before a swim (or bath or shower), you will need to cover your PD catheter with a special plastic dressing, which you will be able to get either from your renal clinic or from your family doctor. After a swim (or bath or shower), you will need to clean the exit site of your catheter and, if possible, also do a fluid exchange.

5. Sexual activity. Most people stay sexually active while on PD. Some people may find it uncomfortable to have sex with the dialysis fluid in, but they can drain it out first and use a new bag afterwards. Patients on APD can have sex either before or after the dialysis starts. The connecting lead for the APD machine is very long and need not restrict you.

6. Stability. As PD takes place continually, all day and all night, people on PD generally feel fairly well most of the time. This is because their bodies do not have to put up with the rise and fall of toxins or fluid levels in the blood experienced by people who are on haemodialysis three times a week.

DELIVERY AND STORAGE OF SUPPLIES

PD is a home-based therapy and so requires regular delivery and storage of supplies. The bags of dialysis fluid come in boxes of two, four or five. So a month's supplies can be as many as 40 boxes. These can be stored in a cupboard under the stairs, a spare bedroom, the shed or even the garage.

Most people receive a delivery of supplies once a month, although patients with very small houses or flats may be able to arrange fortnightly deliveries. The people who deliver the supplies deliver to many other dialysis patients, and are specially recruited and trained to go into patients' homes. They will move the supplies to exactly where a patient wants them, and will even move boxes around so that fluid from previous deliveries gets used before the new stock.

POSSIBLE PROBLEMS WITH PD

PD is not always entirely trouble-free. Patients may experience various emotional and physical problems:

Emotional problems

PD requires commitment as people have to do dialysis every day. Some patients do not like the way PD affects their appearance. The abdomen may appear slightly rounded. Keeping fit and doing exercises to strengthen the abdominal muscles will help.

The PD catheter can also cause body image problems. Some people find this very difficult to cope with and may worry that it might put off a sexual partner. (*See Chapter 15* for more information about the psychological aspects of kidney failure.)

Physical problems

1. Fluid overload. PD can remove the build-up of excess fluid that healthy kidneys would usually remove. However, in some people, either PD doesn't remove enough fluid or the person has taken too much fluid in, meaning that they will have fluid overload. This can cause swelling of the ankles and breathlessness. Fluid overload can be improved by using stronger dialysis fluid and by drinking less.

2. Backache. Some PD patients find that the dialysis fluid in their abdomen is uncomfortable and can cause backache.

3. Poor drainage. This can have a number of causes. The PD catheter may become blocked with a substance called fibrin, which is a form of protein. This looks like tiny strands of cotton wool and is completely harmless. It is easily cleared by squeezing the tubing. Alternatively, a nurse will be able to clear the catheter by injecting a de-clotting agent, called heparin, down the catheter. This is a simple procedure and will not need an operation. Another common reason for poor drainage is constipation. This can cause the bowels to press against the catheter and make the dialysis fluid drain very slowly. So it is very important to avoid constipation, perhaps by taking regular laxatives.

4. Leaks. Dialsysis fluid can leak from around the tube if the catheter has not been given time to heal before it is used. If a leaking catheter is 'rested' (not used for dialysis) for 2–4 weeks, it will usually 'seal up' again, and become watertight.

5. Hernias. A hernia occurs when a wall of muscle weakens and lets an organ or tissue bulge through from inside. If an existing hernia is noticed by the surgeon during an operation to insert a PD catheter, it will be repaired during the same operation to stop it causing problems in the future. If a hernia occurs at a later date, it should also be repaired. This may require a 4–6 week period of haemodialysis while the operation heals.

6. Infection. All dialysis patients are prone to infections. Although they can usually be treated with antibiotics, it is better to avoid getting an infection in the first place. This can be achieved by strict attention to hygiene. Care is needed both with personal hygiene and when the dialysis is performed.

An infection of the peritoneum is called peritonitis. It is usually caused by germs getting into the dialysis fluid when the exchange is done. This can happen if a person touches the connection between the bag of fluid and the catheter. Being scrupulously clean during the exchange procedure can reduce the risk. While many people on PD never get an infection, some will get one once every couple of years, some will get one more frequently.

Occasionally, a patient may get several attacks of peritonitis in a row. The doctor may then decide that an operation to replace the PD catheter is needed straight away.

Another type of infection, called an exit site infection, may also occur. This causes a red tender area around the exit site (the point where the PD catheter comes out through the skin). Keeping the catheter taped down to the skin will help reduce the risk of an exit site infection. Keeping the exit site clean and dry will also help reduce the risk of an infection. Many people will also use an antibiotic cream around the exit site every day. This has been proven to significantly reduce the risk of infection.

Exit site infections respond well to antibiotics, usually given as tablets or creams.

Occasionally, an exit site infection spreads down the catheter 'tunnel' (the route taken by the catheter through the abdominal wall). If antibiotics are not effective, an operation to remove the catheter will be necessary. It is usually possible to insert a new catheter at the same operation.

KEY FACTS

1 In peritoneal dialysis (PD), the process of dialysis takes place inside the patient's abdomen.

2 PD is suitable for most people with ERF.

3 Your own peritoneum (abdominal lining) acts as the dialysis membrane.

4 There are two types of PD: CAPD (a manual technique that you do) and APD (an automated technique that a machine does). In the UK, 60% of patients have CAPD, and 40% have APD.

5 Dialysis fluid is drained into the peritoneal cavity, left there until dialysis has taken place, and is then drained out.

6 You, will be trained to do the dialysis yourself, in your own home.

7 One advantage of PD is the independence it gives you. It enables you to take control of your own life and look after yourself at home.

8 You will need storage space in your home to accommodate supplies of dialysis fluid.

9 Problems with PD include infections and hernias, although many patients don't experience any problems.

10 HAEMODIALYSIS

This chapter describes haemodialysis, which is a form of dialysis used to treat people with chronic kidney failure in a hospital, satellite unit, or at home.

INTRODUCTION

Haemodialysis treatment became available in the 1960s. The main difference between haemodialysis and peritoneal dialysis or PD (see *Chapter 9*) – is that the process of dialysis (see *Chapter 8*) takes place intermittently, outside the body, using a machine for just a few hours a day, or overnight on fewer nights per week.

Currently, about 4% of haemodialysis patients have their dialysis at home, 70% are treated in a hospital and the other 26% go to a 'satellite dialysis unit'. People who go to the hospital or a satellite unit have their dialysis on average three times a week for about four hours each time. Home-based haemodialysis, however, is usually done more frequently – up to six times a week for just a few hours a day or fewer times a week, overnight.

HOW DOES HAEMODIALYSIS WORK?

Haemodialysis is a treatment that takes over some of the work normally done by the kidneys. It removes the waste products of food (toxin clearance, see *Chapter 2*), and removes excess water from the body (see *Chapter 3*).

The basic principles of dialysis are explained in detail in *Chapter 8*. Briefly, both types of dialysis use a special liquid (called the dialysis fluid, dialysis solution or dialysate) and a membrane (called the dialysis membrane) to do some of the work of the kidneys.

In haemodialysis, the process of dialysis occurs in an artificial filter through a machine. This machine is called a dialysis machine or kidney machine (see *top diagram, page 69*). Blood from the patient is pumped through the machine so that dialysis can take place.

The filtering unit called the dialyser or artificial kidney (see *bottom diagram, page 69*) is a cylinder that contains thousands of very small hollow tubes. Each of the tubes is made from very thin plastic, which acts as the dialysis membrane. The patient's blood is pumped through the middle of the tubes. Meanwhile, the machine pumps dialysis fluid around the outside of the tubes. The process of dialysis takes place through microscopic holes in the tubes. Various substances and water can easily pass through the holes, but blood cells cannot.

During dialysis, waste products (such as creatinine and urea) pass from the blood into the dialysis fluid. They do this by a process called diffusion, by which substances pass from a stronger to a weaker solution (see *page 54*). Meanwhile, other substances that are needed by the body (such as bicarbonate and calcium) can be supplied to them from the dialysis fluid. Again, it is diffusion (now working in the opposite direction) that makes this possible.

The second main function of the kidneys (and therefore of dialysis) is to remove water. In haemodialysis, it is the action of the dialysis machine that removes the water. The machine applies a sucking pressure, or negative pressure that draws water out of the blood and into the dialysis fluid. This process is known as ultrafiltration (see also *page 54*) or 'u…f…ing'. Instructions about the amount of water to be removed and the rate of ultrafiltration are entered into the machine at the start of each dialysis session, depending on how much excecss water the patient has to lose.

HOW IS HAEMODIALYSIS DONE?

During haemodialysis blood is taken from the body and pumped around a dialysis machine and through a dialyser. In the dialyser, waste products and excess water pass from the blood into the dialysis fluid. The cleansed blood is then returned to the body at the same rate at which it is removed. Meanwhile, the 'used' dialysis fluid (full of waste products and extra water) is pumped out of the dialysis machine and down the drain.

HOSPITAL AND SATELLITE-BASED HAEMODIALYSIS

Patients who opt to have their dialysis in the renal unit usually have their treatment three times a week for about four hours each session. The exact length of the sessions will depend on the amount of waste that an individual patient produces; bigger people generally need longer dialysis sessions than smaller people. However, if a patient has a lot of fluid to remove, they may need to spend extra time on the machine.

The schedule is fixed by the hospital so, typically, a patient will be given a 'slot' for their treatment such as every Monday, Wednesday and Friday between 8 AM and 12 PM, or every Tuesday, Thursday and Saturday between 1 PM and 5 PM for example.

Nurses are present during the treatment and will usually set up the machine, insert the needles and attach the patient to the machine. They will also monitor patients during the dialysis and be on hand should any problems arise.

Many kidney units now encourage their more able patients to become involved in their own care. This may mean simply having patients check their own blood pressure before dialysis; but it may go as far as teaching patients to put themselves on to, and take themselves off, the dialysis machine.

Satellite haemodialysis takes place away from the main hospital, in a 'satellite unit'. At the satellite unit, patients are treated by relatively few nurses. The patients generally do some of the dialysis preparation themselves. This allows patients to feel more in control of their treatment than is often possible in hospital-based units.

Satellite units can be more convenient for patients as they tend to be nearer to residential areas than many hospital buildings, making them more accessible by car or public transport. Parking is usually easier. It may also be possible to arrange haemodialysis sessions after normal working hours.

HOME HAEMODIALYSIS

The main advantage of having haemodialysis at home is that patients aren't restricted by the fixed schedules of the hospital. They are able to do their dialysis at a time that suits them and their family. While home haemodialysis (HHD) can be carried out three times a week in the same way as hospital-based haemodialysis, there is now some evidence that overnight haemodialysis (also known as nocturnal haemodialysis) and more frequent (5–6 times a week) HHD has many health benefits for patients. There are reports that people who do more frequent or longer hours on haemodialysis need fewer medications.

Training for home haemodialysis takes up to six weeks, and patients and an assistant (usually a family member) learn all aspects of the treatment. They won't be expected to go home on dialysis until they feel completely confident to do so. Like PD patients who are also on dialysis at home, haemodialysis patients have access to specialist support on the phone 24 hours a day. They will also have regular home and clinic visits to make sure that everything is working well.

Requirements for home haemodialysis

Successful home haemodialysis requires patients to have no problems with their vascular access. Patients must also be able to learn to do the dialysis, and be able to solve any problems that might occur during a dialysis session.

Some renal units also recommend that home haemodialysis patients also have a 'helper' present during their dialysis sessions.

People who have their haemodialysis at home will need an area in which to perform their treatment. Many people use a spare room, or put the machine in a convenient area of their home.

Haemodialysis machines generally require specially treated water and so adaptations are needed to be made to the home. The renal unit will organise this, although this might take time to set up. Some new machines have an integrated water treatment system, making them more convenient.

Home haemodialysis requires regular delivery and storage of supplies. These can be stored in a cupboard under the stairs, a spare bedroom, the shed or even the garage. Most patients will receive a delivery of haemodialysis supplies every month, although patients who just have home haemodialysis three times a week may have deliveries less frequently. The people who bring the supplies deliver to many other dialysis patients, and are specially recruited and trained to go into patients' homes. They will move the supplies to exactly where a patient wants them, and will even move boxes around so that fluid from previous deliveries gets used before the new stock.

DIFFERENT DIALYSERS AND MACHINES

There are many sorts of dialyser available, and different renal units tend to have their own preferences. The membrane inside the dialyser can be made from different materials and some have a bigger surface area available for dialysis. Although the dialysers may look quite different from one another, the way in which they

How a dialysis (kidney) machine works

1 Blood comes from the arm

2 Blood is pumped through the machine

3 Heparin (a drug to prevent clotting) is added to the blood

4 Blood enters the dialyser. Dialysis fluid with treated water (a) enters the dialyser, and wastes are taken away to a drain (b)

5 Blood passes through a bubble trap

6 Blood goes back to the arm

A dialyser (artificial kidney)

work is the same. The same applies to dialysis machines. Manufacturers opt for different colour schemes and shapes. Also, different machines display information in different ways, but they all tell much the same story. Some newer haemodialysis machines are designed specifically for home haemodialysis. They are smaller than conventional machines and some are portable, so patients can travel without needing to organise haemodialysis at another renal unit.

'ACCESS' TO THE BLOODSTREAM

The term 'access' soon becomes familiar to patients on haemodialysis. It refers to the method by which access is gained to the bloodstream so that dialysis can take place.

During haemodialysis, large quantities of blood must be rapidly removed from the body, and (at the same time) just as rapidly returned to it. Therefore, in most cases, access has two 'sides'. One of these (called the 'arterial side') is used to take blood out of the patient's body. The other (called the 'venous side') is used to return blood to the patient after dialysis.

There are two main types of access:

- a fistula, which is formed from the patient's own blood vessels by joining a vein to an artery (see below); and

- a dialysis catheter, which is usually a double-barrelled plastic tube (see page 71).

FISTULAS

The usual form of access for haemodialysis is the arteriovenous fistula or AVF (often simply called a fistula). Fistulas are the preferred method of access compared to catheters because they do not use any plastic, and so are less likely to become infected. A fistula will generally last longer than a catheter (see page 71).

Fistulas are made by a surgeon in a small operation, which may be performed under a general or a local anaesthetic. In this operation (see diagram, opposite), a vein (a blood vessel that carries blood back to the heart) is joined to an artery (a blood vessel that carries blood away from the heart). This can be done under the skin, usually at either the wrist or the elbow.

The blood pressure in arteries is always higher than the blood pressure in veins. When a fistula is formed, blood from the artery flows into the vein, and causes it to enlarge a little. Once the fistula has 'matured' (i.e. grown) it will be ready for dialysis. This usually takes about 6 weeks. If a patient is approaching the need for haemodialysis reasonably slowly, it will be possible to plan ahead and create the fistula at the best time. There will be a best time. If the fistula is made too early, it will have to wait to be used which is not ideal. But if it is too late, it will not be ready in time when the patient really does need dialysis. Most doctors would advise creating the fistula when the creatinine level is around 300–350 mol/l, or the eGFR is 15–20 mls/min. This is usually 6 months to a year before dialysis becomes necessary and gives time for the operation to be repeated if unsuccessful first time.

Fistulas are not always successful. In a UK research study in 2008, success rates for wrist fistulas were 49, 41 and 32% at 6, 12 and 24 months, respectively; and 57, 51 and 38% for elbow fistulas. To put it another way, most last 2–3 years. As this study suggests, brachial fistulas (fistulas at the elbow) are more successful than radial fistulas (at the wrist) – i.e. more likely to develop into something that can be used for dialysis. However, although the success rate is lower for a radial fistula than for a brachial one, doctors will usually try a radial fistula first. This is because once a person has had a brachial fistula, they cannot then have a radial one. But if they have had a radial fistula first, and it ceases to work, it may still be possible for them to have a brachial fistula created.

A fistula

1 Normal vein

a Artery takes blood to the arm and hand
b Vein takes blood from the hand and arm

2 Vein diversion

c A diversion of the vein is formed, linking it to the artery in the forearm

3 Vein thickens

d The vein thickens beyond the link, and can now be used as a fistula

Whenever a fistula is used for haemodialysis, a local anaesthetic may be applied to the skin and then two large needles are inserted into the fistula. These needles provide access to the bloodstream for dialysis, and are removed at the end of the session.

The creation of a fistula means some blood that would otherwise have gone to the hand (or arm) in the artery used for the fistula, instead bypasses the hand or arm and goes up the fistula. This does not normally cause any problems. However, occasionally, the hand or arm becomes cold and painful because of the blood that is 'stolen' from it by the fistula. This is called steal syndrome. Severe steal syndrome may mean that the fistula has to be 'tied off' – i.e. permanently blocked off – by a surgeon during another small operation.

Steal syndrome is more common in brachial (elbow) fistulas, which is a disadvantage of that type of fistula, even though the initial success rate is high.

When a fistula is touched, a buzzing sensation is felt. This is known as a bruit (pronounced 'broo-ee'). Patients with fistulas are advised to check for the buzz every day. They should do this gently as fistulas can be fragile.

If there is no buzz when a fistula is touched, this probably means that the fistula has become blocked by a blood clot. Often this occurs at night and is caused by accidentally sleeping on the fistula arm. If no buzz can be felt, it is important to contact the hospital as soon as possible as it may be possible to clear the clot and save the fistula.

HAVING 'DIFFICULT ACCESS'

Being told they have 'difficult access' is something no dialysis patient wants to hear. The usual scenario is that a fistula stops working and a dialysis catheter becomes necessary.

DIALYSIS CATHETERS

A haemodialysis catheter is a plastic tube, usually with two separate barrels, one for removing blood from the body, and the other for returning it after dialysis. The catheter, which needs to be half in and half out of the body, is inserted during a short operation. This operation may be performed under either a general or a local anaesthetic. The catheter is inserted into a large vein either at the side of the neck, under the collar bone, or at the top of the leg next to the groin (see *diagram, page 72*). Names sometimes used for catheters in these different places are a 'jugular line' (at the side of the neck), a 'subclavian line' (under the collar bone), and a 'femoral line' (in the groin). It can be used for haemodialysis almost immediately after it is inserted.

Dialysis catheters may be temporary or semi-permanent. Temporary catheters are often used while patients are waiting for a fistula to be created. Other patients – particularly those with diabetes – have blood vessels that are not strong enough for a fistula, and will need a semi-permanent catheter for haemodialysis access.

Semi-permanent catheters are tunnelled deeper under the skin than temporary catheters. They also have small cuffs around them, just under the skin, to help keep them in place, and to help keep germs out of the body. Semi-permanent catheters also tend to be softer and more flexible than most temporary catheters. These tend to be used when a patient's fistula has stopped working.

After each dialysis session, saline (salt dissolved in water) is injected into the line to remove any blood. The inside of the catheter may then be filled with a drug called heparin. Heparin stops the formation of blood clots, which could block the catheter. This keeps the catheter clear of clots between dialysis sessions. In some hospitals, the dialysis catheter is injected with antibiotics after use to prevent infections. Between dialysis sessions, patients are asked to keep their catheter clean and dry, and to ensure that it has a dressing on it at all times.

Without access, patients who are treated by haemodialysis cannot dialyse. It is therefore very important that everyone – doctors, nurses and patients – all treat catheters and fistulas with great care.

OTHER TYPES OF ACCESS

There are other types of access available, which are used when the two main types (double-barrelled catheters and fistulas) no longer work. This usually happens in patients with fragile blood vessels.

Entry positions for haemodialysis catheter lines

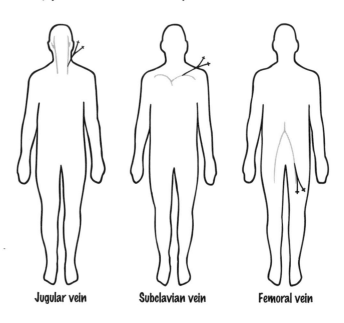

Jugular vein   Subclavian vein   Femoral vein

Grafts. A graft is a plastic connecting tube that joins an artery to a vein, inside the patient's arm or leg. (It is therefore different from a fistula, in which the patient's artery and vein are joined directly without a plastic connector.) The graft must be inserted by a surgeon during an operation. Grafts are made of a special self-sealing material (for example, Gortex) through which dialysis needles can be inserted. A graft can be used within days of being inserted.

Single-barrelled catheters. It is sometimes necessary to use a single-barrelled catheter. This is inserted into the same sites that would have been used for a double-barrelled catheter. If a single-barrelled catheter is used, it is necessary to use single-needle dialysis principles (see below).

SINGLE-NEEDLE DIALYSIS

It is also possible to do haemodialysis using a single needle to remove and return the blood (rather than the two needles used for 'normal' dialysis). The single needle is inserted into a fistula or a graft. Alternatively, a single-barrelled catheter can be used. The blood-flow through the 'single needle' is continuously reversed. So some blood is removed and sent towards the dialyser, and then some of the 'cleaned blood' is returned to the patient. This 'stop-start' dialysis isn't as effective as conventional (two-needle) haemodialysis and so isn't used that often. Single-needle dialysis is sometimes used for patients who have developing fistulas or grafts, or if a patient's fistula never enlarges properly.

WHO CAN BE TREATED BY HAEMODIALYSIS?

Almost all patients with established renal failure (ERF) can be treated by haemodialysis. The only real requirements are:

- It must be possible to gain good access to a patient's bloodstream (see *page 70*). (Access can be a particular problem for kidney patients who have diabetes, see *page 75*.)

- Patients must be able to withstand major changes in blood pressure and toxin levels. (Most people have no problems with this, but some patients with heart problems may have complications.)

LIVING WITH HAEMODIALYSIS

The need to do haemodialysis regularly has an inevitable effect on lifestyle. Having to make frequent trips to the hospital can be an irritation, and may interfere with family or work life. Home haemodialysis may be less disruptive, but still involves a long-term regular commitment to the treatment by the patient and other members of the family.

If you are on haemodialysis, there may be practicalities that restrict your holiday choices. Holidays can sometimes be difficult to arrange because you will need to find a dialysis centre that is willing to treat you while you are away from home.

Some haemodialysis patients need a semi-permanent catheter to provide access, and they may feel unhappy about the effect this has on their appearance. However, the more usual form of access for haemodialysis is the fistula, which is less visible. (See *Chapter 15* for more information about the psychological aspects of kidney failure.)

The patient and doctor may have different perceptions of what a 'good fistula' is. What the doctor sees as being 'an excellent, working fistula' may appear to the patient as 'a great, ugly bulbous thing that needs to be hidden'.

POSSIBLE PROBLEMS DURING HAEMODIALYSIS

Haemodialysis is not always entirely trouble-free. Patients may experience various psychological and physical problems:

PSYCHOLOGICAL PROBLEMS

Life on haemodialysis can feel restricted. Keeping a restricted diet and fluid intake can be difficult. However, making sure you don't get fluid overloaded between dialysis sessions will certainly help your health. It is also important to talk regularly to the nurses and dietitians, to see whether your blood test results are OK. You may need to restrict some things that you eat, for example. if they contain salt, phosphate or potassium. If you take an interest in your diet and ask for advice, you will feel more in control and you will probably be healthier. Though sometimes you may wonder what is OK to eat! (See *Chapter 14* for more information about eating well with kidney failure.)

Some patients have body image problems with their haemodialysis access. A plastic catheter or fistula can be unslightly. (See Chapter 15 for more information about the psychological aspects of kidney failure.)

PHYSICAL PROBLEMS
Fluid overload

Haemodialysis can remove the build-up of excess fluid that healthy kidneys would usually remove. However, as haemodialysis (carried out in a hospital or satellite unit) is not done every day, the build-up of fluid in the body in between each dialysis session can be excessive. This can cause a number of problems. Firstly, fluid overload puts additional pressure onto the heart muscle, and if a patient is regularly very fluid overloaded, the heart muscle becomes damaged. Secondly, the effects of removing a lot of excess fluid during one dialysis session can cause the patient to have a rapid fall in blood pressure (sometimes called 'crashing'). This can cause fainting, vomiting, cramps, temporary loss of vision, chest pain, fatigue and irritability.

The best way to avoid problems caused by rapid blood pressure changes during haemodialysis is for patients to stick to recommended fluid intake limits. For most haemodialysis patients, the recommended daily fluid intake is about 1 litre of fluid. (PD patients can usually have 1.5 litres.)

Intermittent treatment

Three times a week, hospital or satellite haemodialysis is a more 'aggressive' form of dialysis than PD or daily home haemodialysis. In hospital or satellite haemodialysis, all the dialysis is crammed into two or three sessions a week, each one lasting only 3–5 hours. In other words, the balloon is let down very quickly. The rapid changes in blood pressure (usually a fall), and in the blood levels of water and body wastes that occur during a haemodialysis session, can make some patients feel quite unwell, either during or after the session.

Hyperkalaemia (excess potassium)

Another problem that may occur between intermittent hospital or satellite haemodialysis sessions is hyperkalaemia – too much potassium in the blood (see also *Chapter 14*). A raised level of potassium in the blood may cause the heart to flutter, and even stop. Hyperkalaemia can be very dangerous. It requires urgent medical treatment, and sometimes immediate dialysis. If you are on haemodialysis and hyperkalaemia is a problem for you, it is likely that your doctor will advise you to be very careful about eating any food that is high in potassium.

Home haemodialysis patients, who do their dialysis more frequenetly than hospital haemodialysis patients, may have less of a problem with hyperkalaemia, as the potassium levels don't have time to build up between the dialysis sessions.

PROBLEMS WITH HAEMODIALYSIS ACCESS

There may also be problems with the different types of haemodialysis access.

As discussed above (*pages 70–72*) the usual type of haemodialysis access is a fistula, and if this works well haemodialysis will be technically easy. However, as was clear from the discussion of 'difficult access' (*page 71*) not all fistulas do work perfectly. Some never develop into a vein that is large enough for the blood flow to be adequate. Some function for months or even years, then suddenly stop working. In either case, a surgeon will then have to make a new fistula (or sometimes a graft) in another part of the body. Unfortunately, there are only a certain number of veins that are suitable to be used in this way. Anyone who needs haemodialysis for a large number of years may eventually run out of suitable veins.

To use a fistula (or graft), it is necessary to insert needles into it at the start of each dialysis session. Even with a local anaesthetic, some patients find this painful. Because of the limited 'life' of fistulas, grafts and dialysis catheters, haemodialysis may eventually become impossible. This can be a particular problem for patients with diabetes mellitus (sugar diabetes).

Dialysis catheters may also cause problems. Some patients find it difficult to cope with their changed body image (see *Chapter 15*). Another problem is that dialysis catheters sometimes stop working because they have become blocked by a blood clot. If a catheter stops working, it will have to be replaced. Again, as for fistulas and grafts, there are only a certain number of veins suitable for plastic tubes. Dialysis catheters are more likely to become infected than either fistulas or grafts.

If a graft becomes infected, this can be very serious. It may be necessary to have another operation to remove the graft.

PROBLEMS FOR PEOPLE WITH DIABETES

Over time, diabetes can cause a person's blood vessels to become very narrow. This can make it almost impossible to form a fistula in some patients. Inserting plastic tubes into the veins can also be very difficult. This is why some doctors recommend PD rather than haemodialysis for kidney patients with diabetes, especially when they first start dialysis.

There is also a fear that the drug heparin, which is normally given during haemodialysis to prevent blood clotting, can cause bleeding at the back of the eye (as well as other sites). Most people with diabetes and kidney failure are prone to this type of bleeding (a condition called diabetic retinopathy), by the time they need dialysis. Diabetic retinopathy can cause blindness. It may therefore be better to avoid having to use heparin.

However, not all doctors think that haemodialysis is inadvisable for this group of kidney patients. Some consider that haemodialysis is just as good as PD, does not worsen vision, and may indeed have some advantages for many people with diabetes.

BLEEDING

Haemodialysis patients may have problems with bleeding either during a dialysis session or, more commonly, after dialysis when the fistula needles are removed. Sometimes bleeding can result from using heparin during dialysis. So most centres now try to use as little heparin as possible, and some people have heparin-free dialysis. To try to stop the bleeding after dialysis, it is common for the heparin to be turned off at least 1 hour before the end of the dialysis session.

INFECTIONS

There is always a risk that a patient will pick up an infection during a dialysis session. Germs may enter the patient's blood either from the haemodialysis access or from the lines of the machine. During sessions of dialysis, fevers often become worse and there may be rigors (shivering attacks).

Infections can usually be treated with antibiotics, but it is better to avoid getting an infection in the first place. This can be achieved by strict attention to hygiene. Care is needed both with personal hygiene and when the dialysis machine and access lines are set up. Fistulas are much less likely to get infected than dialysis catheters.

Patients may sometimes develop an infection where the haemodialysis catheter comes out from under the skin. This is called an exit site infection, and causes the area around the catheter to become sore and inflamed. Most exit site infections respond well to antibiotics.

The inside of the catheter can also become infected. This is called a line infection, and can make you very unwell, causing fever and rigors. If you develop a line infection, your catheter may be removed and replaced after the fever has settled. But if you don't have many other possible sites for access, it may be left in until you have had 3 or more infections. A very bad infection will mean it has to be taken out immediately even if there are few other options. Temporary catheters are more likely to become infected than semi-permanent ones, and for this reason temporary catheters should be replaced after about three weeks of use even if they are not obviously infected. This helps to prevent line infections.

KEY FACTS

1 In haemodialysis, the process of dialysis takes place inside a machine.

2 Haemodialysis is suitable for most people with kidney failure and can be done at home, in the hospital renal unit or at a local 'satellite' dialysis unit.

3 In a haemodialysis session, blood is taken from the body, pumped into the dialysis machine, cleaned by an artificial kidney (dialyser), and pumped back into the body.

4 Hospital or satellite-based haemodialysis is usually done two or three times a week, each session lasting 3–5 hours. Home-based haemodialysis is usually done more frequently, either at night or for short periods (about two hours) every day.

5 If you are going to do haemodialysis, you will need direct access to your bloodstream. The usual types of access are a fistula (made by joining a vein to an artery) or a dialysis catheter.

6 Some people feel sick or dizzy during a haemodialysis session. This is usually due to the rapid removal of water and toxins, which results in a rapid drop in blood pressure.

7 If you are on haemodialysis, you will need to control the amount of fluid you drink more strictly than if you were on PD.

8 Fistulas, grafts and dialysis catheters all have a limited life. In practice, this means that haemodialysis may eventually become impossible for some people.

11 TRANSPLANTATION

This is the first of three chapters that provide information about kidney transplants. It covers the issues and the various procedures that are necessary before a patient can have the operation.

INTRODUCTION

A successful kidney transplant is a more effective treatment for kidney failure than either peritoneal dialysis (see *Chapter 9*) or haemodialysis (see *Chapter 10*). This is because a well-functioning transplanted kidney can do all the jobs of the kidney, whereas dialysis only really does a couple of these jobs. However, not all patients are suitable for transplantation, and not all suitable patients are suitable all the time.

Also, before a transplant can take place, it is necessary to find an appropriate donor kidney, which may not be easy.

THE BENEFITS

A kidney transplant can deliver the best quality of life to people with ERF. There is no doubt that for the right patient at the right time, a transplant is the best treatment option. A 'good' transplant provides about 60% of the function of two normal kidneys (compared with only about 5% from either type of dialysis). Then the blood creatinine level will be under 150 µmol/l (i.e. a stable transplant patient with a well-functioning kidney will still have chronic kidney failure at Stage 2 or 3).

The most obvious advantage of a transplant to people with kidney failure is freedom from dialysis. If a transplant works well, dialysis becomes a thing of the past. There are also no particular fluid or dietary restrictions after a transplant. Erythropoietin and calcium tablets, such as Calcichew, can usually be stopped. Most people who have had a transplant feel better and have more energy than they did on dialysis. They are better able to cope with a job, and many find their sex lives improve. Women are more likely to get pregnant and have a healthy baby.

WHO CAN HAVE A TRANSPLANT?

Up to 40% of patients with kidney failure are suitable for a transplant, provided a suitable donor kidney can be found (see *page 79*). Patients who will probably not be considered suitable include anyone with serious heart or lung disease, or with many types of cancer.

Most kidney units do not have an age limit for kidney transplantation. Patients are considered on merit (i.e. their suitability for a transplant) rather than age. However, having said that, most units would think very seriously before transplanting a patient over 70 years old.

Doctors do not believe that transplanting an older patient 'wastes' a kidney that a younger person would get 'more benefit' from. The main reason for limiting transplants among older patients is that they often do not tolerate the operation very well. Also, the drugs that are needed after a transplant (see *page 99*) are often too strong for older patients.

NEW KIDNEYS AND OLD DISEASES

Patients who are having kidney transplants sometimes worry that the original cause of their kidney failure might make the new kidney fail too, but this is very unusual. An exception, however, is where the original kidneys failed because the patient had a condition called focal and segmental glomulerosclerosis (FSGS). This is a type of glomerulonephritis, and it comes back in around 20% of patients who have had it before. Patients who have lost one kidney due to recurrent FSGS have a 50% chance of losing another one.

There are a few other types of glomerulonephritis and related conditions that may also come back and affect the transplanted kidney. These include mesangiocapillary glomerulonephritis (variable, depending on type), Goodpasture's disease (25%), haemolytic uraemic syndrome (less than 25%), membranous nephropathy (less than 25%), IgA nephropathy (10%), Henoch-Schönlein purpura (10%), and lupus nephritis (1%). But these conditions, if they do recur, do not necessarily lead to loss of the kidney. However, if FSGS or one of these other conditions were to recur in two consecutive kidneys (causing their failure) doctors would be unlikely to recommend a third transplant.

Patients who are affected by any of these conditions, should ask their doctor about the likelihood of the original disease recurring, and damaging a kidney transplant.

DO YOU HAVE TO BE ON DIALYSIS FIRST?

Many renal units will talk to patients about having a transplant during the pre-dialysis period as it may be possible to organise a transplant, particularly if a living donor can be found, before the patient needs to start dialysis. This is usually done when the blood creatinine is about 400 µmol/l (micromoles per litre of blood) and the eGFR 15 mls/minute – i.e. at the end of Stage 4

kidney disease, which is about six months before dialysis will be needed. Also, if someone has a transplant that is failing, they may be put onto the list at this same point, and given a new kidney before they have to go back on dialysis.

The national waiting list is for what is known as a deceased donor transplant (*see page 80*). This type of transplant uses a kidney that has been removed from someone who has died; 64% of the kidneys transplanted in the UK come from this source. The remaining 36% are what are known as living related transplants or LRTs, and living unrelated transplants or LURTs (*see page 90*). For some patients, the possibility of obtaining a transplant kidney from a living donor will be the best chance of having a transplant operation before dialysis is needed.

Given that it is possible for people with kidney failure to be given a transplant before they need dialysis, you may wonder why patients cannot do this. The reason is that most doctors think that because there is such a shortage of kidneys for transplantation, it is better if patients all around the UK start waiting for a kidney at an equivalent time point, i.e. when they start dialysis. This makes it fair for everyone.

However, some kidney units are undoubtedly better organised in terms of transplantation than others. So some units do carry out more transplants before dialysis. Some units also make more effort to obtain kidneys than others and do more transplants, and some units are keener on living transplants than others. For all these reasons, patients in some units may wait less time for a transplant; and be more likely to have a transplant before they need dialysis, than is usual in other units.

You have a right to ask the doctors, nurses or managers about the performance of your unit. You may want to ask them how many transplant operations they do, and how long (on average) these transplanted kidneys last. How many of the transplants they carry out are of kidneys from living donors? Can you have a transplant from a living donor before you need to go onto dialysis? You have a right to know the answers to these questions, and the data are all on the NHS Blood and Transplant website (*see page 163* for address). You will find that performance does vary quite considerably around the UK.

FINDING A SUITABLE KIDNEY

For a kidney transplant to be successful, it is better that the tissues of the new kidney are fairly similar (i.e. 'matched') to the patient's original kidney. If the new kidney is not a good enough match, the patient's immune system (natural defence system) will be more likely to attack and reject it. (See *page 97* for a description of the rejection process.)

Before a suitable kidney can be looked for, it is necessary for patients to have a number of tests. The most important of these are to find out the patient's blood group and type tissue (see *below*). The results will then be checked against the results of similar tests carried out either on an available kidney, or on a relative or other person who is considering donating one of their kidneys to the patient.

MATCHING THE BLOOD GROUP

The blood group is an inherited characteristic of red blood cells. It stays the same throughout your life. There are four main blood groups. These groups are called A, B, AB and O. Group O is the most common, followed by group A, then B then AB – except in Asian patients, in whom group B is more common than A.

The blood group that you belong to depends on whether or not you have certain substances called antigens (types of protein) in your body. Two different antigens – called A and B – determine a person's blood group. If you have these antigens, they will be on the outer surface of all your cells, not just on your blood

cells. If you have only antigen A, your blood group is A. If you have only antigen B, your blood group is B. If you have both antigen A and antigen B, your blood group is AB. If you have neither of these antigens, your blood group is O.

The function of the blood group antigens is not known exactly. They may act as a 'friendly face' for the cells, so the rest of the body can recognise the cells as their own, and leave them alone. A person's immune system will attack any cells that have a foreign antigen. This means a patient can only be given a transplant kidney if the patient's and donor's blood groups are matched as follows:

Patient	Donor
Group O	Group O
Group A	Group A or group O
Group B	Group B or group O
Group AB	Any group (O, A, B, or AB)

MATCHING THE TISSUE TYPE

The principle of matching for tissue type is similar to that for matching for blood group. Again, the patient and the donor kidney or potential donor are matched using a blood test. The tissue typing test shows a person's genetic make-up (a type of 'genetic fingerprint').

The tissue type is an inherited set of characteristics (antigens) on the surface of most cells. It stays the same throughout your life. You have only one tissue type (just as you only have one blood group), but your tissue type is made up of six different tissue type characteristics.

There are three main sorts of tissue type characteristic, called A, B and DR. Everyone has two of each (one from each parent) – making six in all. Just to make it more complicated, there are many different types of A, B and DR characteristic. In fact there are 20 or more different versions of each A, B and DR characteristic. This means that there are hundreds of different possible tissue types. So, for example, a tissue type could be A1/A2, B7/B8, DR2/DR3.

As there are so many possible tissue types, matching tissue types is a little more complicated than matching blood groups. However, basically the more of these that are the same for both patient and donor kidney, the better will be the chances that the transplant kidney will work.

Given the large number of tissue type possibilities, it is very unusual to get an exact match (known as a '6 out of 6 match' or 'full-house match') between a patient and donor. Most units will offer a transplant if the patient and donor have three or more of the six tissue type characteristics in common, and there is at least one DR match. In terms of tissue typing, it is more important that the DR characteristics are matched than the A or B types. So, for example, a transplant might be offered in the following situation:

Patient:	**A1**/A2	**B7**/B8	**DR2**/DR3
Donor:	**A1**/A3	**B7**/B12	**DR2**/DR7

As the A1, B7 and DR2 characteristics are the same in this example. It would be called a '3 out of 6 match, including one DR match'.

The more characteristics that match the better. So a '6 out of 6 match' is better than a '3 out of 6 match'. The better the match, the more likely it is that the body will accept the kidney 'as its own', and not try to reject it.

Unfortunately, it cannot be guaranteed that even a '6 out of 6' match will not be rejected. This is because the blood group and tissue type are not the only cell surface characteristics that are important. However, these other important characteristics have not yet all been identified. Tissue-type matching is less important for transplants from living donors where a 1 out of 6 match may be satisfactory (see *page 86*).

TESTING FOR VIRUSES

Before a patient can be put forward for a transplant, they will have to be tested for various viruses. These include HIV (the virus that causes AIDS), hepatitis B, hepatitis C and cytomegalovirus (CMV). It is important to test for these viruses because they may be dormant ('sleeping', causing no symptoms) in a patient's body. After the transplant, they may be 'woken up' and cause illness. This is especially true of CMV.

Patients who refuse to have any of these tests, such as the HIV test, will not be able to have a transplant. If a patient has one of the viruses, it does not mean that they will not get a transplant, it just means the doctors will have to be more careful.

OTHER TESTS FOR TRANSPLANT SUITABILITY

Other tests are also necessary before a patient can have a transplant. These include an electrocardiogram (ECG, an electric recording of the heart beat), a chest X-ray, and sometimes an echocardiogram (ECHO, a sound-wave picture of the heart) and an 'exercise test' (a test in which the patient has to walk on a moving walkway, to test their fitness, and stress the heart). Some kidney units also insist that kidney patients who have diabetes also have a cardiac catheter test (a special X-ray picture of the heart). This cardiac test has some risk, causing death in 1 in 1,000 patients.

If results of all these tests are satisfactory, the patient can then be put on the national waiting list (see *page 82*) for a deceased donor transplant, or considered for a possible transplant from a living donor.

DECEASED DONOR TRANSPLANTS (AND HOW LONG THEY LAST)

The term 'deceased donor transplant' is used to describe a transplant kidney that has been removed from someone who has died. In 2008, 64% of transplant kidneys in the UK came from this source, and current follow-up studies indicate that 93% (about 9 out of 10) are working after the first year (see also *page 86*).

But what do all these percentages and fractions mean for you? In other words, how long will *your* kidney last? Well, it's difficult to say, but on average, a deceased donor transplant will last more than 10 years. Yours may last 5 minutes or 20 years, or it may not work at all. But the average is 10 years. Doctors have still not been able to make deceased donor kidney transplants last a very long time.

WHERE DO DECEASED DONOR KIDNEYS COME FROM?

Most of these donors have been killed in car accidents or died from a stroke, and have been on a life support machine (ventilator) in an intensive care unit. The ventilator is breathing for them. Their kidneys can be removed after the person has been diagnosed 'brain dead'. This means the part of the brain called the brainstem, which controls breathing, has permanently stopped working, and the person is legally certified as dead. The doctors then record this in the medical notes.

Once brainstem death is diagnosed, this is irreversible, and the person's ability to breathe for themselves will not return. An individual who is brainstem dead cannot remain on a life support machine indefinitely, as their heart will stop relatively soon.

If the person on the life support machine is not going to be a donor, their machine would be switched off at this point. If they are going to be a donor, their kidneys for donation are usually removed immediately after the donor's heart has stopped beating, which occurs shortly after the life support machine has been switched off. For this reason, these donors are sometimes called 'deceased brain dead'.

DECEASED CARDIAC DEAD DONORS

Because of the shortage of donors, some kidney units are obtaining transplant kidneys from people who have died up to 30 minutes previously. These donors – called deceased cardiac dead (or asystolic) donors – are people who have died very suddenly, sometimes from a heart attack. Their hearts have stopped beating, and they are dead. They have not necessarily been put on a life support machine.

Patients who have kidneys from deceased cardiac dead donors are quite likely to have a period of dialysis after the transplant. This does not normally affect the long-term results.

Patients who are offered a transplant can ask whether it is from a cardiac dead or brain dead donor. They have a right to know this, even though they will not be told any other details about the donor. After receiving a deceased donor kidney, patients may write to the donor's family, via the transplant co-ordinator, if they wish, but it is essential that both donor and recipient remain anonymous. Patients should feel free to discuss these issues with their transplant co-ordinator after the transplant.

If someone is on the national waiting list (see *below*) for a deceased donor kidney, they can still ask a relative, partner or friend to give them a kidney. These living transplants are described more fully in *Chapter 12*. It is not as important to have a well-matched transplant if the donor is a living person (see *page 86*).

XENOTRANSPLANTATION

The term 'xenotransplantation' refers to the possibility of using organs (such as kidneys) taken from animals (especially pigs) for transplantation into humans. A certain amount of research has been done in this area, but the problems are currently considered to be too great. One major concern is the risk of passing on animal viruses to humans.

STEM CELL 'KIDNEYS'

Research is also being carried out to see if kidneys can be grown or repaired using stem cells. These are very simple cells taken from an adult (or human fetus) that can be programmed to grow into more mature (kidney-like) cells.

Although this research has received considerable publicity, and might change the face of kidney failure in years to come, it is doubtful it will help people with kidney failure in the near future.

THE TRANSPLANT WAITING LIST

At present, not enough deceased donor kidneys are donated to meet the demand. Changes in seat-belt laws and improvements in medicine mean that fewer people now die from the accidents or illnesses that would have made them suitable donors.

So people who are waiting for a deceased donor kidney are put on to a waiting list. Their details, including their blood group and tissue type, are put onto a national computer at NHS Blood and Transplant in Bristol. When surgeons remove two kidneys from a patient who has died, this organisation finds the most suitable patient for each kidney – either locally or in the rest of the country.

A nationally agreed 'scoring system' decides where the kidneys go. It is based on a combination of blood group and tissue type matching, and the length of time the patient has been on the waiting list, and some other factors. Even though it is as fair as it can be, some patients are disadvantaged – especially Asian people. This is partly because Asian people have different blood groups from white people, and there are fewer suitable Asian donors. It is particularly important therefore for Asian patients to find a living donor in their family, as they may have to wait a very long time to get a deceased donor kidney in the UK.

The waiting list works on the basis of finding the 'right' dialysis patient for the 'right' kidney, when one becomes available. It does not work on a 'first-come, first-served' basis. Transplants are allocated to the patient who is the best match for the kidney in terms of blood group and tissue type. In other words, the patient does not join a queue, knowing that his or her name will come up after a reasonably fixed time. It is not really a waiting list, more of a register. The average waiting time for a transplant is about 3 years. It is important to note that this is an average: it can be 2 days, or 20 years – or never.

It may sometimes be necessary to take a patient off the transplant list. This may be done, for example, if someone develops a serious infection or a heart problem, or if they need a major operation. The decision is not made lightly. Any patient whose name is removed from the list should be told about the decision, and informed whether removal from the list is temporary or permanent.

Patients who are unsure whether or not they are 'on the list' should ask their kidney doctor or nurse and then ask them for proof in writing. They can also ask their unit staff to inform them if their name is ever taken off the waiting list.

BEING READY FOR A TRANSPLANT

Patients who are on the waiting list for a transplant will not be given very much notice that a kidney is available for them. So they need to be prepared to go to the hospital at short notice. Some patients are given a 'bleep' so that they can be contacted more easily. It may be sensible to leave your mobile phone on 24 hours a day. If you take a holiday outside the UK, you may miss a call when a kidney becomes available.

When patients are on the transplant waiting list, it is largely up to them to make themselves contactable at all times, day and night. If a patient cannot be found, the kidney will be offered to someone else. When a patient 'gets the call', they should go to the hospital at once and not have anything to eat or drink (in preparation for the anaesthetic).

TESTS BEFORE THE OPERATION

Patients called in to the hospital for a transplant are not guaranteed to receive it. Before the operation can go ahead, it is necessary to check that the patient is well enough to have the operation, and that they will not reject the transplant kidney:

1. Physical examination. The patient is first given a thorough physical examination by a doctor. The purpose of this is to check that it is safe to proceed with the operation. For example, if a patient has a heavy cold, it may considered too much of a risk for them to have an anaesthetic. If the patient 'fails' this assessment, they will be sent home, and put back on the waiting list.

2. The cross-match. This test is the final hurdle before the operation. The cross-match is a blood test that checks the patient has no antibodies (substances that normally help the body to fight infection) that would react with the donor kidney. High levels of such antibodies in the blood mean that the new kidney is likely to be rejected as soon as it is put into the patient, even if it seems a good match.

A cross-match is done by mixing a sample of the patient's blood with blood cells from the donor. If there is no reaction (i.e. if the patient's blood does not start attacking the donor's cells), it is assumed that the patient will be less likely to reject the new kidney when it is transplanted. This is called a negative cross-match, and means that the operation can go ahead.

If the cross-match is positive (i.e. there is a reaction between the patient's blood and the donor's cells), the patient will be sent home and put back on the waiting list. This can be very disappointing, but it is much better to return to dialysis for a while than to be given a kidney that doesn't work, and which may make the recipient extremely ill.

THE TRANSPLANT OPERATION

Undergoing an operation to have a kidney transplanted is a major procedure, and afterwards all patients have to take certain medicines and other precautions for the rest of their lives. This applies whether the transplanted kidney was from a deceased donor or from a living donor. More details about the operation itself, and life after transplantation, are given in *Chapter 13*.

KEY FACTS

1 For the right patient at the right time, a transplant is the best treatment for kidney failure.

2 If a transplant works well, you will be totally free from dialysis, able to eat and drink normally and continue working. Your sex life may also improve.

3 Suitability for a transplant is more important than age. Up to 40% of patients with kidney failure may be suitable to receive a transplant.

4 Transplants are matched to individual patients in terms of blood group and tissue type.

5 Transplant kidneys come from three sources: deceased donor transplants, living related transplants and living unrelated transplants.

6 The transplant waiting list works on the basis of finding the 'right' kidney for the 'right' person – i.e. patients do not join a queue.

7 Patients have to wait on the transplant waiting list for an average of about 3 years. Asian or Black patients may have to wait longer, so should certainly consider a living transplant if a suitable donor is available.

8 Patients who are called into hospital to receive a kidney transplant need to undergo a series of tests before the operation to make sure the kidney is suitable for them.

12 LIVING DONOR TRANSPLANTATION

In this chapter we discuss the issues surrounding living donor transplantation, the procedures and processes involved, the benefits of this type of transplant, and some of the possible problems.

INTRODUCTION

The first successful kidney transplant was a living donor transplant. It was performed on 23 December 1954 by Joseph Murray and his team at the Peter Bent Brigham Hospital, Boston, USA. A kidney was removed from one man and transplanted into his genetically identical twin brother.

In the UK, the majority of kidneys for transplantation are donated by people who have died (deceased donor transplants). However, a significant proportion (in 2008, this was 36% in the UK) are donated from a relative or someone close to the person who has kidney failure. Human beings do not need two kidneys – quite why we have a 'spare one' is not known. The loss of one kidney will not usually cause any harm to the donor, providing the other one is healthy and functioning. The proportion of living transplants is increasing *every* year. In some UK units, it now accounts for 60% or more of all transplant operations. In countries, such as Japan, where deceased donor transplantation is almost unheard of for cultural reasons, living transplant offers the only real option to coming off or avoiding dialysis.

A transplant from a living donor can have many benefits. For most patients, the possibility of a transplant kidney from a living donor will be the best chance of

having a transplant operation before dialysis is needed. If a loved one is donating a kidney, the whole transplant procedure will be planned, and both donor and recipient are usually well prepared for the operation.

However, there are risks with the procedure. Just as with a deceased donor transplant, the kidney may not work – in fact, 1 in 30 living transplants are not working a year after the transplant operation. So it is worth considering the emotional aspects of living transplantation before embarking on the process. Both you and the donor need to talk about the possibility of complications following the operation, and how you might feel if the transplant doesn't work.

A growing number of units now have a transplant co-ordinator whose main job is to organise living transplants. This is part of the reason why these transplants are becoming more common. Anyone who is on the list for a deceased donor transplant can have a live transplant if they have a suitable donor.

THE BENEFITS (AND HOW LONG THEY LAST)

Accepting a kidney from a loved one means that the wait for a transplant may be shorter than the wait for a deceased donor transplant. In some circumstances, the transplant may take place before you need to start dialysis. The transplant operation can also be planned, on a date which is suitable for everyone involved, whereas deceased donor transplants often happen at very short notice.

A kidney from a live donor is likely to function for longer than a deceased donor kidney. In 2008, in the UK, 97% of living donor transplants were still working after the first year (that is more than 19 out of 20), 88% after 5 years and 68% at 10 years. This is in contrast to only 93% of deceased donor transplants at one year (just under 19 out of 20), 83% at 5 years, and 64% at 10 years after a transplant.

These statistics are all very well, but anyone considering accepting a kidney from a living donor will want to know how long a living transplant will last for *them*. As with a deceased donor kidney (see *page 80*), any individual living donor transplant may last 5 minutes or 20 years, or indeed it may not work at all. But, on average, a living donor transplant will last 15 years (that is 5 years of 'extra kidney life' when compared to a deceased donor kidney).

No one really knows why a living donor transplant usually lasts longer than a deceased donor one – particularly since the tissue type is usually less well matched to that of the person receiving the transplant. Certainly, a kidney being transplanted from a living donor is usually of better quality than a deceased donor kidney.

This is because living donors are carefully screened for any diseases that might affect their kidneys, such as hypertension or diabetes. The donor's kidneys are also checked to make sure that they function perfectly, and are not likely to fail in the future. Also, a living transplant is more likely to be done before dialysis because it is often one of the first avenues the consultant will 'explore' when a patient is first diagnosed. So the patient does not have to experience the stress of dialysis on blood pressure and the heart.

Also, the time in which the kidney is outside a human body after it has been removed from the donor (i.e. 'still fresh') – called the cold ischaemia time – seems to be a crucial factor. This is less than one hour for a live transplant, but 12–36 hours (the average is 20 hours) for a deceased donor transplant. The benefits of transplanting the kidney as soon as possible after it is removed from the donor seem to be much more important than other issues such as tissue type for the success of the transplant.

A living donor transplant may improve the relationship between donor and recipient, as there is a common bond between the two. However, relationships can be complicated and this may not always be the case. There is also some evidence to suggest that the recipient of a living donor transplant is more likely to take the medication required after the transplant, perhaps because the recipient feels more of a responsibility towards the new kidney.

If your kidney failure is diagnosed at an early stage, you could be considered for live kidney transplant up to 6 months before you need dialysis. At this point your creatinine level is likely to be about 400 µmol/l (micromoles per litre of blood). If you already have a transplant that is starting to fail, you could have a live transplant before you need to return to dialysis. But this is up to your own kidney unit's individual policy.

PATIENT SURVIVAL AFTER LIVING DONOR TRANSPLANTS

There is some evidence that patients who have a living donor transplant will live longer than those receiving deceased donor transplants – having a 99%, 95% and 89% chance of being alive at one, five and 10 years after the transplant, if the transplant is still working. These results are not directly comparable to deceased donor transplants where there is a 96%, 87% and 68% chance for a patient with a deceased donor transplants at the same time points. Nonetheless, there is a tendency for patients who have had a living donor transplant to live longer.

SURVIVAL AFTER TRANSPLANTS: COMPARISON TO DIALYSIS

These survival rates may not seem that good (either for living donor or deceased donor transplants), as most patients have their transplant when they are quite young. But these numbers should be compared with what would happen if the patient stayed on dialysis. For example, 20–25% of patients die within one year of starting dialysis. This is a not an entirely fair comparison, as transplant patients are generally younger than many people on dialysis and so would be expected to live longer. While doctors may not necessarily believe transplants are more likely than dialysis to improve survival for patients with kidney failure, there is general agreement that they can offer a better quality of life.

DECEASED OR LIVING DONOR TRANSPLANT – WHICH IS BEST?

It is difficult to give firm advice about which is the 'best' type of transplant, even though there are clear medical benefits of a living donor transplant to the recipient. These benefits, outlined above, are in terms of the likelihood of both the kidney working and the patient being alive at 5 and 10 years after a transplant. There are significant risks to the donor. Nonetheless, it is the view of the authors that if both sides are willing, and understand and accept the risks, then it is 'better' for most patients that their first transplant is a living donor transplant. This is especially important in families, such as Asian and Black families, where a suitable deceased donor kidney is likely to be harder to come by. If this first transplant ever fails, they could then have another living donor transplant, or a deceased donor transplant.

In the end, it is up to each donor and recipient pair to make the decision, having taken in the type of information put forward in this chapter, and discussed this with their doctors and the rest of their family.

WHO CAN DONATE A KIDNEY?

Almost anyone can donate a kidney to a loved one. The best donor is an identical twin, as the tissue type is identical. Unfortunately, most people do not have an identical twin waiting to give them a kidney. A kidney from a non-identical twin may also be suitable, but again, few patients have non-identical twins. If a kidney patient has a friend, partner or relative who is at least 16 years old, healthy, and willing to give them a kidney, they should speak to the transplant co-ordinator (or other senior nurse or doctor) at their unit.

The most suitable donor is usually a father, mother, brother, sister, son or daughter, but other more distant relatives may be suitable – uncle, aunt, nephew, niece, cousin, grandparent or grandchild. In fact, the donor does not necessarily have to be a blood relative. The patient's wife, husband, partner or close friend may also be suitable. About 50% of people, blood relatives or otherwise (if they are fit), may be suitable to donate a kidney to any given patient.

As human beings do not need two kidneys to be healthy, the donor is unlikely to come to any harm by losing a kidney. But even if a kidney comes from a loved one, it is important both donor and the patient understand that the kidney is not guaranteed to work.

However, there are some situations where it would not be possible for a living person to donate a kidney. These include potential donors with the following conditions:

- HIV or AIDS-related infection;
- hepatitis B or C infection;
- major heart or breathing problems;
- diabetes (either type);

- significant kidney disease;
- most cancers;
- very high blood pressure;
- intravenous drug abuse;
- extreme obesity;
- pregnancy;
- having only one kidney;
- evidence of financial or non-financial coercion;
- inability of a potential donor to give informed consent; or
- age below 16 years.

In addition, doctors would think very seriously before allowing anyone to donate a kidney if any of the following applied:

- age over 70 years;
- age below 18 years;
- intellectual impairment but able to give informed consent;
- mild obesity;
- family history of diabetes;
- psychiatric disorders; or
- mild high blood pressure. (i.e. needing more than one blood pressure tablet).

WHICH DONOR?

Although it may be difficult for some patients to find a suitable living donor, others can find they get a number of offers from family and friends when they are told they will need a transplant to treat their kidney failure. Each potential living donor will be assessed for their medical suitability to donate a kidney, and to ensure they are well before, during and after the operation. If more than one person is a suitable donor, it can be difficult to decide which one to accept a kidney from.

But if a patient has a parent and a brother or sister, both of whom are willing (and able) to donate, it might be 'better' to accept the kidney from the parent now, and then 'keep' the sibling's kidney for later in life, if the first transplant ever fails. However, there are no hard and fast rules. The situation will vary between different patients; each individual will have different relationships with the various members of their family circle, and will not necessarily feel closest to their nearest blood relative.

There is no evidence that a woman of child-bearing age (provided she is not actually pregnant at the time) will be at any more risk than anyone else who is offering to be a donor. Nor is there any evidence that it will affect her chance of getting pregnant, or put a future pregnancy at risk.

WHO WILL DO THE ASKING?

It is up to kidney patients to ask their friends or family to see if they are willing to donate a kidney. Doctors will not usually ask a patient's loved ones for them, but they will talk to anybody who is willing to donate a kidney.

TESTS FOR THE DONOR

As with a living donor transplant, the first and perhaps the most important test, to see if the potential transplant might work, is a simple blood test to find out the blood group of the donor. Usually, if the patient's blood group and the donor's blood group are not compatible (according to the rules outlined on *page 79*), no further tests will be carried out. The transplant is unlikely to go ahead, so the transplant tests will be stopped.

Some units have now introduced a technique called antibody incompatible transplantation (or 'desensitisation') which makes it possible for a patient to have a successful transplant when a donor is in the 'wrong' group. (More information about transplants using this technique is given below.) If your transplant unit does not do this type of transplant, you can be referred to another transplant centre.

If the test is OK, blood samples will be taken to test the donor's liver and kidney function. If these prove satisfactory, the next stage of the screening process can then go ahead.

The donor will need to have a thorough medical examination. This is usually done by two separate doctors – a kidney doctor (usually a different one from the doctor responsible for the patient), and the surgeon who will perform the operation. The doctors will check to make sure that the donor has a normal blood pressure. If their blood pressure is found to be high, the doctors will monitor it for 24 hours – this is because it may only be high at certain times of the day or in certain circumstances. In some cases, the doctors may still agree to go ahead with the transplant, even if the donor has high blood pressure, just as long as it is well controlled using only one type of blood pressure tablet.

An ultrasound scan will then be used to make sure that the donor has two kidneys, and that both are functioning equally well. The function of the individual kidneys can be assessed by a test such as nuclear medicine test (see page 48). Each kidney should be providing 50% of the total kidney function. It is no good if one kidney is undertaking 70% of the work while the other kidney only does 30% of the work. If the surgeon then removed the kidney that did 70% of the work, this could be disastrous for the donor.

The potential donor will also have an ECG (a heart trace, see page 152) and a chest X-ray to ensure there are no problems with their heart or breathing. They may also be given an exercise tolerance test to see how their heart reacts under light exercise.

Blood tests will be carried out for infections such as HIV and hepatitis B and C. Blood samples will also be used to test the donor's genetic compatibility with the recipient (tissue type). This is necessary for all live related transplants so that the genetic relationship between donor and recipient can be proven. Tissue matching is also undertaken in live unrelated transplantation to find out if the donor and recipient are well matched. However, as discussed above (page 79), close matching is not necessary in living transplants.

In addition, there will also be a cross-match test (as in deceased donor transplantation) between donor and recipient. As with deceased transplantation, if the cross-match is negative, this means the transplant work-up can continue, but if the cross-match is positive, the transplant cannot normally go ahead. However, sometimes an antibody incompatible transplant (see below) can get around this problem.

Most units also carry out a psychological assessment of both donor and recipient. This is to make sure that both are happy about the procedure, and the effects it may have on them and their families. The psychologist will make sure that both people are able to cope if the transplant fails or if anything happens to either the donor or the recipient.

Finally, to help the surgeons decide which kidney (left or right) to remove, the blood vessels to each kidney must be examined using either a type of computed tomography (CT) scan that takes a special look at the blood vessels to the kidneys (a CT angiogram), or a magnetic resonance angiogram (MRA).

TESTS FOR THE RECIPIENT

These are the same as those outlined in Chapter 11 (pages 82–3).

ANTIBODY INCOMPATIBLE TRANSPLANT

Some recipients will have high levels of antibody to a potential donor. The recipient may also have the 'wrong' (i.e. incompatible) blood group, tissue type, or both. These situations used to make transplantation impossible, as both would lead to the recipient's immune system attacking (rejecting) the new kidney. But the situation has changed with the development of a technique called antibody incompatible transplantation (or 'desensitisation'). This is carried out in a few transplant centres in the UK. It involves using immuno-suppression that is stronger than normal; using a dialysis-like process called plasmapharesis and strong drugs. Initial results have been good, with kidney survival almost as good as with 'normal' living transplantation.

LIVING UNRELATED TRANSPLANTS

Most living donor transplants are performed using kidneys from people who are related to each other, such as genetically related family members. These are called living related transplants (LRTs).

However, an increasing number of live kidney transplants use the organs from people who are not genetically related to each other, although they do have a 'relationship' with each other. This could either be through marriage, co-habitation or a long-standing friendship. Whatever the circumstances, before any living donor transplant can go ahead, the relationship must be proven. These are called living unrelated transplants (LURTs).

If the donor and the recipient are from the same family, the relationship can be proved from blood samples. If the relationship is an emotional one (husband, wife, partner or friend), it must be proved in other ways. Each case must be reported to the Human Tissue Authority (HTA), an authority regulated by the Department of Health. Under the Human Tissue Act, passed in 2004, the HTA, whose role is to ensure that the kidney is being donated freely and for no other reason than to benefit the recipient's health, must approve all transplants from living donors following an assessment by an Independent Assessor appointed by the Authority. This is necessary whether or not the donor and the

person receiving the kidney are related to each other.

The information the donor and the recipient will need to provide for this assessment will vary according to the nature of their relationship. The Authority will advise you what will be relevant in your case.

PAIRED AND POOLED DONATION

An exciting development that has been introduced since the Human Tissue Act in 2004 is that of 'pairing' and 'pooling' donated kidneys. If a person who needs a new kidney has a family member or close friend who is willing to donate a kidney to them, all will not necessarily be straightforward. For example, incompatible blood groups or tissue types could result in serious problems. One way to address this is by using antibody incompatible transplantation, described above. But paired and pooled donation offers a realistic alternative. Paired donation allows people in this situation to be matched up with another donor and recipient in the same situation, under the watchful eye of the HTA.

Sometimes, more than two donors and two recipients will be involved in the swap (pooled donation), but each recipient will benefit from a transplant that they would not otherwise have been able to have.

Local transplant centres will assess whether people are suitable to be put forward for paired or pooled donation. If so, their details will be put on to a national register where they can be matched to a compatible pair. Donor and recipient operations are planned to happen at the same time so that organs can be exchanged at the same time.

ALTRUISTIC DONATION

The 2004 Human Tissue Act made it legal for a person to donate a kidney to a stranger. This is called an altruistic donation. Some of these altruistic transplants are now happening. The donor must go through the same checks as a donor who is known to the recipient.

BUYING AND SELLING ORGANS

In the UK, it is illegal to buy or sell kidneys for transplant. There must be no pressure put on to any potential donor to donate, or recipient to accept.

Even though it is illegal to offer payment to enable the live transplant to take place, it is legal for the donor to be repaid reasonable costs incurred due to travelling (even from abroad) or loss of earnings. This facility is included in the Human Tissue Act (2004). The renal social worker should know how to obtain this money from the Health Authority or Primary Care Trust.

BEING OFFERED A DECEASED DONOR TRANSPLANT WHILE PLANNING A LIVING DONOR TRANSPLANT

If you are on the deceased donor waiting list, and having the necessary tests for a living transplant, you may be lucky enough to be offered an organ from a deceased donor. You will then have to make the difficult decision whether or not to accept the organ. This decision will be made harder by the fact that it is possible that the living transplant may have better results. If the deceased donor organ is not a good match, or it is not a particularly 'good' organ, it may be better to say 'no', and proceed with your living transplant. But ultimately, the decision is a personal one that you will need to discuss with your family, your donor and your doctors.

PREPARATION FOR A LIVING DONOR TRANSPLANT

The length of time it takes to prepare the donor and recipient for a living donor kidney transplant can vary from one unit to another, depending upon a variety of factors:

- The process will be quicker if there is a full-time dedicated living donor transplant co-ordinator.

- The process may be delayed if it is necessary for either donor or recipient to have additional pre-transplant tests as a result of initial screening.

- If the donor is not a blood relative of the recipient, it will be necessary to contact the HTA (see above) for permission to carry out the operation. This usually takes about two weeks, athough getting all the necessary information together can take considerably longer.

On average, it can take around 3–6 months to prepare for a living donor transplant. Sometimes, the time is deliberately long so as to give both parties sufficient time for careful consideration.

It is important that the donor allows for time off work before the transplant as well as after, so that the relevant tests can all be done.

REMOVING THE KIDNEY FROM THE DONOR

There are two ways a live kidney can be donated, either by open surgery, or laparoscopically (using keyhole surgery). The removal of a kidney is called a nephrectomy:

1. Open nephrectomy. Open surgery is the more usual method of removing the kidney. The surgeon makes a cut from the middle point of the side of the chest to the side of the abdomen. Part of a rib may also need to be removed. This method leaves a much larger scar than keyhole surgery. It also takes longer for the donor to recover after the operation. However, using conventional surgery significantly reduces the risk of complications during the operation.

2. Laparoscopic nephrectomy. Some kidney units remove the kidney using keyhole surgery. A small cut is made above the pubic hairline (a 'bikini' or 'low bikini' cut). The kidney is located and removed with the help of a small camera that helps the surgeon to see inside the body without cutting the patient right open. The benefit of this procedure is that the patient has a smaller scar and a quicker recovery time. But there are some disadvantages. There is an increased risk of complications, such as potential damage to the kidney being donated.

Whichever method is used to remove the kidney, the surgeon takes great care not to damage the organ in any way. The surgeon also removes the blood vessels and tubes surrounding the kidney, as they will be used for the recipient.

If the kidney is removed using laparoscopic nephrectomy, the donor will be in hospital for about 3–5 days, but after open surgery this could be 6–9 days.

How soon the donor returns to work will depend on the type of work and their general fitness before the operation. If the work is physically demanding, the donor will probably need a longer recovery time than someone who has sedentary work.

If the kidney is donated by laparoscopic nephrectomy, the donor can probably return to work within 3–4 weeks of the operation. With open surgery, it is advisable to remain off work for about 12 weeks.

RISKS TO THE DONOR

Although any surgical procedure carries with it a small risk, the risks to a healthy donor should be minimal if all the pre-operative tests have been carried out. The donor should be aware, however, that the more invasive tests (such as the angiogram) do themselves carry some risk. Anyone who donates a kidney will be seen regularly after the operation. Most units recommend kidney donors should be seen by a kidney specialist every year for life. There is some evidence to suggest that kidney donors live longer than other people on average – nobody knows why this might be so. It may be that they 'look after themselves' better when they know they have lost a part of their body.

There will be some pain and discomfort after the operation, which should get better after a few days. One in 25 patients, however, get long-term pain in the site of the wound. This can usually be controlled by injections given from time to time.

There is usually a 10–20% rise in the donor's creatinine level after losing a kidney.

Some donors may experience protein in their urine (proteinuria) after the operation, and about 10% of all donors may develop high blood pressure. This is the same as the incidence of high blood pressure within the general population.

There is a 1 in 3000 chance of the donor dying during or after the operation. This is similar to the risk of any major operation.

A more common and major problem of donating a kidney to a loved one is the potential emotional upset if a living donor transplant fails at an early stage.

RISKS TO THE RECIPIENT

For the recipient, a live kidney transplant operation carries the same risks it would do for a deceased donor transplant (see page 97).

Also (as mentioned on page 78) some patients may find their original disease, especially a type of glomerulo-nephritis called focal and segmental glomerulonephritis (FSGS), may return in a transplanted kidney. This is a problem in both deceased donor and living donor transplants, but will not necessarily cause the transplant to fail.

REJECTION

Unless the live transplant has come from a genetically identical donor (an identical twin), there will be a risk of rejecting the kidney. Around 40% of patients may experience rejection at some point in the first year after a transplant (not necessarily leading to loss of the kidney). This is about the same as the risk for people who have had a deceased donor transplant. It means that it is very important for patients to take their immuno-suppressant medication very carefully, to help avoid this problem. More information about rejection and immuno-suppressant medication is given in the following chapter.

CONCLUSION

Living donor transplants are becoming more common in the UK, but there is still a large shortfall in the number of kidneys available. Hopefully, with better awareness of the higher success rate of living donor transplants, the number will continue to rise.

KEY FACTS

1 Although the majority of kidneys transplanted in the UK are from people who have died, around 36% are given by a living relative, partner or friend of the patient.

2 All would-be donors will be carefully assessed to ensure they are fit enough to donate a kidney. Nonetheless, there are risks to both the donor and recipient.

3 Most live donors are related to the patient (LRTs), but an increasing number of kidneys are now being given by partners or friends (LURTs).

4 Live unrelated transplants (LURTs) cannot take place without authorisation from the Human Tissue Authority (HTA).

5 The HTA also makes it possible to donate a kidney to a stranger for purely altruistic reasons.

6 Benefits of living donor transplants include shorter waiting times and the potential for advance planning. The kidneys are likely to last longer than kidneys from a deceased donor, and the patient also may have a better chance of living longer after a living donor transplant than after a deceased donor transplant.

7 Two new techniques have been developed to enable transplants to go ahead when recipient and donor are incompatible. These are called antibody incompatible transplantation and paired donation.

8 It is illegal to buy or sell kidneys for a transplant in the UK.

9 If you have a living donor transplant, the risk that your body will reject the new kidney is still there, as for any other transplant patient. So you, too, will have to take immuno-suppressant drugs very carefully, for the rest of your life.

13 THE TRANSPLANT OPERATION AND AFTER

This chapter describes what happens during a kidney transplant operation, and what to expect afterwards. The importance of continuing treatment, and possible side effects of drugs, are discussed.

INTRODUCTION

Transplanting a kidney is a straightforward operation, with a good success rate. The principles have not changed much since the 1950s, when the first kidney transplants were being pioneered in America. After a transplant, patients will need to take drugs daily for the rest of their lives. If a transplant fails, patients can go back to dialysis or possibly have another transplant.

THE TRANSPLANT OPERATION

An operation to transplant a kidney requires a general anaesthetic and lasts about 2–3 hours. The surgeon makes a diagonal incision (cut) into the abdomen, on the right or the left, below the navel (see *page 96, diagram 1*).

The patient's own kidneys are usually left in place. The transplant kidney is placed lower down in the abdomen, just above the groin (see *page 96, diagram 2*). The transplant kidney has its own artery (to take blood to it), vein (to take blood from it) and ureter (to take urine to the bladder).

The artery belonging to the new kidney is attached to the patient's main artery supplying blood to the leg on that side of the body. The vein belonging to the new

kidney is attached to the main vein carrying blood from that leg. These leg blood vessels are big enough to be able to send blood to and from the new kidney without affecting the blood supply to the leg. The transplant kidney's ureter is attached to the patient's own bladder. A small plastic pipe (called a double J stent) is usually inserted into the ureter (see *page 96, diagram 3*) to help prevent the ureter from becoming blocked after the operation. At the end of the operation, the patient's abdomen is closed with stitches.

POST-OPERATIVE TUBES

Patients waking up from the anaesthetic after the transplant operation, will find they will have several tubes coming out of them. These will include:

- a urinary catheter (a tube into the bladder);

- a central venous pressure (CVP) line (which is placed under the collar bone or in the side of the neck, and measures the pressure of blood inside the heart);

- an intravenous drip in the arm (to give the patient fluid and drugs if necessary); and, probably,

- one or more surgical drains coming out of the abdomen (to drain off any fluid that gathers around the kidney after the operation).

These tubes will be removed one by one over the next few days. The urinary catheter is usually left in place for five days or more. The double J stent is usually removed during a small operation (under local or general anaesthetic) about three months after the transplant. PD patients may also have their catheter removed at the same time. Some haemodialysis patients find their fistula stops working at some stage after the transplant. This does not matter, provided the transplant is working well.

AFTER THE OPERATION

The first few days after the operation are critical, and patients are monitored very closely. Particular attention is paid to blood pressure, fluid intake and urine output. Most patients are able to drink and eat small amounts and also to sit out of bed the day after the operation.

Patients will have their blood creatinine level measured every day. This shows whether or not the transplant kidney is working. The amount of urine that the new kidney makes is not a reliable indicator, as people who have just had a transplant may produce a large volume of urine that does not contain many toxins. In about one third of kidney transplant patients (more if the kidney has come from a cardiac dead donor – see page 81), the kidney does not produce any urine in the first few days (and sometimes weeks) after the transplant. This does not mean that the transplant will never work. If the transplant does not work at the start, patients will need to continue dialysis and play a waiting game until the kidney starts working.

- **A 'good transplant' is one that is working well after one year, not two weeks.**

Patients will usually stay in hospital for about two weeks. After leaving hospital, they will need to go to the clinic very frequently for many months, initially 2–3 times per week, then once a week, then once every two weeks, and so on. When the doctors are satisfied that the kidney is working well, the patient's appointments may be extended to once every three months or so.

It usually takes 3–6 months for patients who have had a kidney transplant to return to normal activities, including work. Transplant patients are recommended not to drive for at least 1 month after the operation. The function of the kidney, and the risk of infection, will not be affected by having sex. However, it is probably best not to resume sexual activity until about four weeks after leaving hospital.

HOW LONG WILL THE TRANSPLANT LAST?

A kidney transplant does not last for ever. The average lifespan of a transplanted kidney is around 10 years for a deceased donor kidney, and about 15 years for a living related transplant. The average for a living unrelated transplant is somewhere between the two. So the 'best' (longest-lasting) kidney transplant is one from a relative, then a friend or partner, then a dead person. There is more information about the length of time you can expect a kidney transplant to last in Chapters 11 and 12.

Another way of looking at how long a transplanted kidney is likely to last is to look at the percentage chance that the kidney will be working at set time points. A transplanted deceased donor kidney has, on average:

- a 93% chance of working one year after the operation;

- a 83% chance of lasting five years; and

- a 64% chance of lasting 10 years or more.

Transplant operation

1 Incision sites (see Note below)
2 New kidney position (right side insertion)
3 Double J stent tube (shown in position)

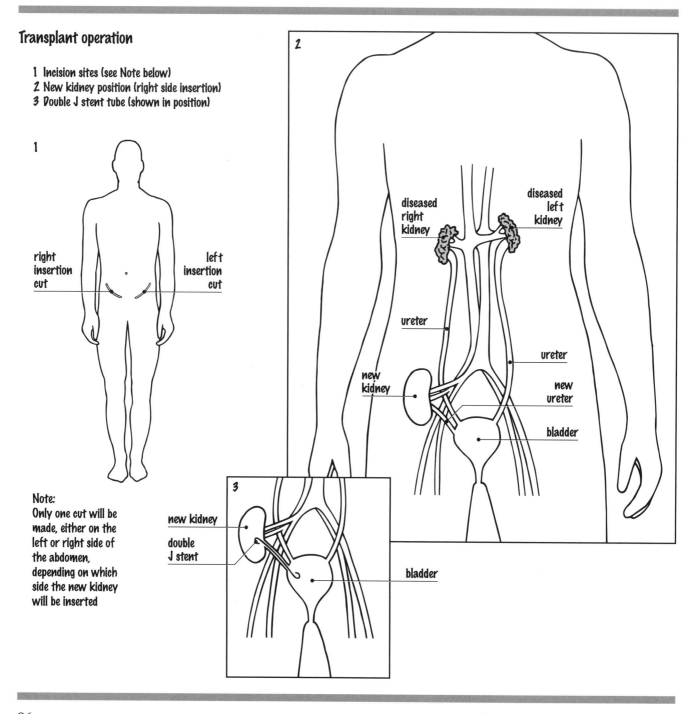

1

right insertion cut

left insertion cut

Note:
Only one cut will be made, either on the left or right side of the abdomen, depending on which side the new kidney will be inserted

2

diseased right kidney

diseased left kidney

ureter

ureter

new kidney

new ureter

bladder

3

new kidney

double J stent

bladder

The chances that a kidney from a cardiac dead donor will still be working at the same time points are similar. The chances that a kidney donated by a living person will be working at these times are higher – on average:

- a 97% chance of working 1 year after the operation;

- a 88% chance of lasting 5 years; and

- a 68% chance of lasting 10 years or more.

Younger patients may need two or more transplants in their lives. If a transplant fails, the patient can restart dialysis, and most can go back on the transplant waiting list.

POSSIBLE PROBLEMS AFTER A TRANSPLANT

Although a transplant is an excellent treatment for most people with ERF, it is not problem-free. Some people who have had a transplant experience a problem called rejection (see *below*). Rejection is part of the reason why transplants do not last for *ever*.

Other problems that a patient may experience after a transplant include drug side effects (see *page 100*), infection (see *page 101*), heart disease (see *page 101*) and cancer (see *page 101*). It must also be repeated that within one year of any transplant, around 5% of patients die.

THE REJECTION PROCESS

'Rejection' means that the patient's body recognises that the transplanted kidney is not 'its own' and tries to 'reject' it from the body. Even when patients and transplant kidneys are apparently 'well matched' (in terms of blood group and tissue type, see *pages 79–80*), some degree of rejection is common. The severity of rejection varies from patient to patient. Rejection may be either acute or chronic (see *page 98*).

The body system that is responsible for the rejection process is called the immune system. The immune system is the body's natural defence system. It is located all over the body, and has many different parts. It includes organs (such as the spleen and appendix), lymph nodes (including the 'glands' in the neck) and specialist white blood cells (called lymphocytes).

The usual task of the immune system is to fight foreign invaders. These include germs (such as bacteria and viruses) and foreign objects (such as splinters or thorns embedded in the skin). The immune system also fights cancer. An individual's immune system does not usually attack that person's own cells because these all have a 'friendly face' (consisting of special proteins called antigens on the outer surface of the cells). The immune system recognises the friendly face and knows to leave the cells alone. Germs and foreign objects do not have this friendly face. Nor do cancer cells, which have developed in an abnormal way.

Normally, the immune system is a 'good thing', as it protects the body from dangerous infections, foreign bodies and cancer. However, after a transplant it can be a 'bad thing'. If the immune system recognises that the new kidney does not have the usual friendly face of the body's own cells, it will become overactive and send lymphocytes to attack (reject) the kidney. The body is actually trying to protect you from the kidney, which it perceives as a danger. Luckily, there are drugs – called immuno-suppressant drugs (see *page 99*) – that can help prevent and treat the rejection process.

ACUTE REJECTION

'Acute' means short term, coming on quickly and needing immediate action. Acute rejection can happen in the first few months (particularly the first few weeks) after a transplant. It is very common – about 40% of patients experience acute rejection in the first year after a transplant. If acute rejection hasn't occurred within 1 year of the operation, then it is unlikely to happen, as long as patients take their drugs correctly. However, if a patient doesn't take their immuno-suppressant drugs, acute rejection can occur at any time. This is why taking these medicines as prescribed, on a regular basis, is so important.

Acute rejection may sometimes cause pain and fever, but usually there are no symptoms. Doctors will suspect that a patient has acute rejection if the blood creatinine level is either not coming down after a transplant, or if it has started to fall and then remains stable or increases again. However, acute rejection is not the only reason why there may be problems with the blood creatinine level after a transplant, and these other possibilities are usually looked for first.

● **Investigations**. Tests that might be performed include an ultrasound scan (see *page 49*). This will show whether the patient's ureter (the tube that takes urine from the kidney to the bladder) is blocked. Other possibilities are specialist scanning techniques called a nuclear medicine scan and a Doppler scan. Either of these will show if there are any problems with the blood supply to the new kidney.

The only way to be sure whether a transplant kidney is being rejected is to do a test called a biopsy. This test is described in more detail on *page 46*. It is common for patients who have had a kidney transplant to have two or more biopsies in the weeks after the operation.

A kidney biopsy is an invasive procedure, and therefore there are some risks involved with having one. For more information about the risks involved, see *page 46*.

● **Treatment.** If the biopsy shows signs of rejection, then the patient will usually be given a high dose of a steroid drug, either prednisolone or methylprednisolone. The drug is given by tablet or intravenous injection, once a day for three days. These short-course, high-dose treatments are called 'pulses'. Very often, this steroid treatment will suppress the rejection process, and the blood creatinine will start to decrease. Occasionally, a patient may need two courses of this (or a similar) drug.

If pulse prednisolone or methylprednisolone does not work, there are various options. For example, one of the immuno-suppressant tablets may be changed to a similar but slightly 'stronger' drug. An example might be tacrolimus replacing ciclosporin (see *pages 100*).

Alternatively, the patient may be given a 5–10 day course of a stronger intravenous injection, such as anti-lymphocyte globulin (ALG), anti-thymocyte globulin (ATG) or orthoclone K T-cell receptor 3 (OKT3) antibody.

These treatments almost always work, and the rejection process goes away. However, all of them can have fairly severe side effects, especially OKT3, which can cause fever, diarrhoea, joint and muscle pain, wheezing, and shortness of breath due to fluid on the lungs (pulmonary oedema).

CHRONIC REJECTION

'Chronic' means long term and of slow onset, not necessarily requiring prompt action. Some doctors think that the term 'chronic rejection' is misleading. The condition it describes is very different from acute rejection. In chronic rejection, there is no real rejection process taking place. The patient's immune system does not attack and reject the transplant kidney in the same way as it does in acute rejection. This is why some doctors call the process 'transplant glomerulopathy' rather than 'rejection'.

Chronic rejection is more like a slow ageing of the new kidney. The cause is uncertain. If it happens, it will usually be more than a year after the transplant operation. Doctors may suspect chronic rejection if a patient's blood creatinine starts to rise slowly after it has been stable for some time. Alternatively, an increasing amount of protein in the urine will be the first sign of chronic rejection. As with acute rejection (see *above*), the only sure way to diagnose the condition is to do a biopsy. There is no treatment for chronic rejection.

The severity of chronic rejection varies. Mild chronic rejection is not usually a problem. However, more severe chronic rejection will eventually lead to failure of the kidney (and therefore a need to go back to dialysis or have another transplant). Chronic rejection may take years to happen, but it is much the most common cause of transplant failure after the first year.

IMMUNO-SUPPRESSANT DRUGS

All patients who have a kidney transplant need to take drugs called immuno-suppressant drugs. As the name 'immuno-suppressant' suggests, the function of these drugs is to suppress the immune system. The aim is to dampen down the immune system sufficiently to stop it rejecting the transplant kidney, while still keeping it active enough to fight infection. Finding the balance can be difficult.

Usually, patients no longer need to continue taking an ESA or calcium tablets after a transplant (see page 32). However, it is vital for them to take two or three different kinds of immuno-suppressant drugs every day. This is because, if they stop taking these drugs, the immune system 'fights back'. If a patient is unable to take these immuno-suppressant drugs, either because they have run out or because they are suffering from diarrhoea or vomiting, they should go to the hospital at once. The immune system does not forget that there is a 'foreign' kidney in the body. It is always waiting for a chance to attack and reject it.

- **If you can't take your immuno-suppressant medicines for 24 hours or more, this will be very serious. Go straight to the hospital where you can get appropriate advice.**

Many other medications (both prescribed and 'over-the-counter') can interact with immuno-suppressant drugs, especially with ciclosporin and tacrolimus, both of which are very 'sensitive' drugs. New medications can cause either of these immuno-suppressants to work too well, increasing toxicity, or work less well, risking rejection. Either of these interactions can cause the creatinine level to go up. So patients should always check with the kidney unit pharmacist, or hospital doctor (not their GP, as it is unfair to expect your GP to have this level of specialist knowledge) before taking *any* new medication. Patients should never assume that just because a medicine or tablet is common and easily available (like aspirin, for example), it is necessarily 'safe' to take if they have a transplant.

THE 'BEST' REGIME OF IMMUNO-SUPPRESSANT DRUGS

There is no best regime of immuno-suppressant drugs. Many drugs are now available. However, doctors are now advised (by NICE – the National Institute for Health and Clinical Excellence) to give patients an injection treatment called basiliximab or daclizumab to suppress their immune system immediately after transplant surgery. This will be given in combination with another drug such as ciclosporin or tacrolimus (FK506). If neither of these prove to be suitable for an individual, alternative drugs, such as sirolimus can be given. One of either azathioprine or mycophenolate mofetil is also usually given. Some people are prescribed steroid drugs such as prednisolone. Other drugs are currently being developed.

If you experience side effects from a particular drug, the drug can be changed for an alternative. Examples might include changing ciclosporin for tacrolimus and vice versa, or azathioprine for mycophenolate mofetil and vice versa.

The choice of drugs is influenced partly by the cost. Also, the long-term side effects of some of the newer drugs are not yet fully understood.

DRUG SIDE EFFECTS

All of the most commonly used immuno-suppressant drugs have their problems:

1. Ciclosporin and tacrolimus. These are the most important drugs used to prevent kidney rejection, and work in a similar way. Unfortunately, if patients are given too much of either, both are toxic (poisonous) to the kidney, this can prevent the transplant from working. This condition is called ciclosporin (or tacrolimus) toxicity. To reduce the risk of problems, patients on either of these will have the amount of the drug in their blood monitored regularly. If problems do occur, these can usually be reversed, either by stopping the drug or reducing the dose. Of course, taking too little of either can increase the risk of rejection. Finding the balance is not easy.

Some patients who take ciclosporin for a long time develop a condition called gum hypertrophy. This is an excessive growth of the gums, which can be unsightly. It is less likely to develop if patients practise good dental hygiene, including regular flossing between the teeth. It the problem becomes severe, the gums can be 'cut back' using a specialist hospital-based dental treatment. Another possible side effect of ciclosporin is excessive growth of hair on the face and body. Tacrolimus does not cause gum swelling or increased hair growth, but can cause hair loss and trembling. Both drugs can cause diabetes, but tacrolimus does so much more often (in up to 30% of patients). If diabetes occurs, it may lead to a lifelong need for insulin injections twice a day.

Both ciclosporin and tacrolimus can also damage the liver and nervous system.

2. Sirolimus. This drug works in a similar way to the above two, but is not so poisonous to the kidney. However, other side effects are seen – especially a very high cholesterol (a type of lipid or fat) level in the blood.

3. Azathioprine and mycophenolate mofetil. The main problem with azathioprine and mycophenolate mofetil is that they can suppress activity in the bone marrow, where blood cells are made. By affecting blood cell production, they can cause a number of serious problems. If too few red blood cells are produced, the patient will suffer from anaemia, causing tiredness. If there are too few white blood cells, the patient will develop a condition called neutropenia. This lack of white blood cells will affect the patient's ability to fight infection. If too few of the blood cells called platelets are produced, the resulting problem is thrombocytopenia, which can cause an increased tendency to bleed.

If you are taking either of these drugs, you may suffer from any or all of the above problems. However, stopping the drug or reducing the dose will normally put matters right. (**NB: this should only be done on advice from your doctor.**)

There are also other side effects. Azathioprine can cause damage to the liver, which will usually be picked up by blood tests. Mycophenolate can cause abdominal pain and diarrhoea.

4. Prednisolone. This drug is a steroid, and, like other steroid drugs, it can cause thinning of the skin (leading to easy bruising) and facial swelling (giving a red and rounded appearance to the face). These problems may lessen if the dose of the drug is reduced.

Like ciclosporin and tacrolimus, prednisolone can also cause diabetes mellitus ('sugar diabetes'). At worst, this might mean that that you would have to take tablets or give yourself insulin injections twice a day. Diabetes can also damage kidneys if it is not well controlled.

A further possible problem with prednisolone is that it can cause crumbling of the joints, especially the hip joints. Pain in either hip, even in the first 3–6 months after a transplant, should be taken seriously. Replacement of one or both hips may become necessary. In the longer term, patients on prednisolone are also at increased risk of thinning of the bones (osteoporosis). Because of this, the vertebrae (bones of the spine) can collapse causing a 'crush fracture'. This can be very painful, as well as reducing your height.

Some doctors try to withdraw steroid tablets after the first 6–12 months because of these side effects on the joints and bones. This usually causes the creatinine to rise by 10 µmol/l (micromoles per litre of blood) or so, which is not usually a problem. But it does carry a very small risk of rejection (or even loss) of the kidney.

INFECTION

Although immuno-suppressant drugs help prevent transplant rejection by making the immune system less efficient, their effect on a patient's ability to fight infections is generally less than might be expected. So people taking immuno-suppressant drugs do not necessarily get one infection after another.

Having said that, there is one infection that is a particular problem after transplantation. It is called cytomegalovirus (CMV) infection. For most people who are not taking immuno-suppressant drugs, CMV is a mild infection that causes a 'flu-like illness. However, in patients who have just received a transplant, CMV infection can be quite a severe illness.

If a transplant patient does ever get CMV, there is a very effective treatment for it. This is called ganciclovir, and is given as a course of injections.

A new virus, the BK virus, has recently been discovered. This can cause the transplanted kidney to function less well, and can also affect the blood. A drug called sidofovir is being used to treat BK virus, although it is not yet known how effective it is. It is given as a course of injections.

HEART DISEASE

Heart attacks and problems with the circulation (such as stroke and reduced blood flow to the legs) are much more common after a transplant. This is partly because of the effects of kidney failure on the circulation before a transplant. It is also due to other new problems after a transplant. These may include high blood pressure, a high cholesterol level in the blood, diabetes (which can start after a transplant, as it is a side effect of many immuno-suppressant drugs) and increased risk of clotting ('thickening') of the blood. The risk of these problems may be reduced if the patient does not smoke, keeps fit, and keeps their weight under control.

If you have had a kidney transplant, you should work with your doctor to keep your blood pressure down (under 120/70 mmHg), your diabetes (if you have it) under control, your cholesterol low (under 5 mmol/l), and perhaps have your blood thinned. This may mean taking more medicines. You may need to take tablets or have insulin injections to control your diabetes. A group of tablets called statins are particularly good at controlling the cholesterol level in the blood. Aspirin can be used to thin the blood, although it will not necessarily be suitable for everyone who has had a kidney transplant.

It is important to ask the doctor why such tablets are not being prescribed, if they are indicated, as having a heart attack or stroke, say five years after a transplant, makes it hardly worth the patient going through such a major operation.

CANCER

One of the functions of the immune system is to fight cancer. By making the immune system less efficient to help prevent transplant rejection, immuno-suppressant drugs unfortunately increase the likelihood of getting some types of cancer. An Australian research study in 2006 has shown that most types of cancer are three times more common in patients with a kidney transplant. Exceptions include breast and prostate cancer.

Exposure to the sun greatly increases the risk of developing skin cancer. In fact, transplant patients are 30–40 times more likely to develop (non-melanoma) skin cancers. The risk for a common type of skin cancer – called squamous cell carcinoma (SCC) – is 80-fold compared to nontransplanted people. Male patients are at particular risk of SCC at sun-exposed sites such as the scalp and the outer ear. All of this makes it very important for people who have had a transplant to use a strong 'sun block' cream to avoid sunburn.

Even though they are very common, provided that skin cancers are diagnosed in good time, they are not usually a major problem. This type of cancer does not usually spread to other parts of the body, and can be easily removed.

LYMPHOMA

A small but significant number (2–5%) of transplant patients develop lymphoma, which is a more serious (leukaemia-like) cancer of the bone marrow and immune system – often within a year of the operation. This is about 10 times the average. It is more common in patients who have had stronger immuno-suppressant drugs. In a majority of patients, it occurs in the first year after transplant. These 'early' cases are particularly serious.

Lymphoma sometimes 'goes away' when the doses of immuno-suppressant drugs are reduced. In more severe cased it has to be treated with high doses of chemotherapy. In some cases, the immuno-suppressant drugs given for the transplant are stopped, which can lead to loss of the kidney. Although these treatments can be successful, 30–50% of people who develop lymphoma after a transplant die within two years of the diagnosis.

KEY FACTS

1 A transplant operation lasts 2-3 hours, and involves staying in hospital for about 2 weeks after the operation.

2 About a third of transplanted kidneys do not work initially, sometimes requiring a short period of dialysis.

3 Up to 40% of patients have at least one episode of acute rejection (of the kidney) after a transplant. These are usually fairly easy to treat.

4 Patients have to take immuno-suppressant drugs daily to prevent their body rejecting a transplant. Not taking them correctly can lead to loss of the kidney. However, these drugs do have side effects.

5 A transplant does not always last for ever. Transplants from living relatives last longest.

6 If a transplant fails, you can go back onto dialysis. Most people can go on to have another transplant.

7 It is important to keep as fit as possible after a transplant. For example, don't smoke, try to keep your weight down, monitor your blood pressure, cholesterol levels and (if you have diabetes) your blood sugar.

8 If you have had a transplant, you will be at greater risk than other people of developing skin cancer, so be extra careful about protecting your skin from the sun. You will also have an increased risk of developing lymphoma, which can sometimes be fatal.

14 EATING WELL

This chapter explains why it is important for people with kidney failure to take care over what they eat. It also describes the different dietary advice that they are likely to be given as their condition and treatment change.

INTRODUCTION

One of the questions most frequently asked by people with kidney disease is, 'Why does the advice given to me about my diet keep changing?' Well, it isn't because the dietitian got it wrong in the first place. The reason is that people's dietary needs change as their condition changes. So, just as drug therapy and other treatments may need to be altered, diet may also need to be revised to stay in line.

HEALTHY EATING GUIDELINES

It is a good idea for all patients with kidney failure – whether pre-dialysis, on dialysis or with a transplant – to follow 'healthy eating guidelines'.

These guidelines are:

- to eat some high-fibre foods (such as wholemeal bread and cereals);
- to eat only moderate amounts of fats (which should be mainly polyunsaturated); and
- to avoid adding 'extra' salt to foods if you have high blood pressure.

WHAT IS 'NUTRITIONAL STATUS'?

The term 'nutritional status' is used by doctors, nurses and dietitians to describe a patient's state of nourishment. A person with a poor nutritional status is not receiving enough of the right kinds of food. There is no single reliable method of measuring nutritional status: there is no nutritional equivalent of the blood creatinine test (see *Chapter 2*).

Doctors, nurses and dietitians usually assess the nutritional status of people with kidney problems by:

- asking how they are feeling;
- asking about the persons's diet (perhaps including asking them to keep a record for a while of everything they eat and drink);
- measuring the level of albumin (a type of protein) in the blood (see *page 44*), as a low level of this is linked to malnutrition;
- measuring the size of the person's muscles; and
- monitoring their body weight.

Research has shown that nutritional status is an important factor in survival. A study of 12,000 haemodialysis patients in the USA showed that patients who had a very low blood albumin when they started dialysis were 17 times more likely to die during the first year of dialysis.

DIETARY PROTEIN AND KIDNEY FAILURE

Protein is an essential nutrient, which enables the body to build muscles, and to repair itself. The main sources of protein in the diet are meat, fish, dairy products and pulses (such as beans and lentils). Everyone – including people with kidney failure – must eat appropriate amounts of protein if they are to avoid serious nutritional problems.

When protein is digested, waste products are formed and enter the blood. One of these wastes is called urea (see page 12). Normal healthy kidneys are quite good at getting rid of urea and other wastes from the blood. However, as kidney failure develops, the kidneys become less and less able to remove wastes from the blood (see Chapter 2). Even so, this does not mean that people with kidney failure should stop eating protein (see below).

DIET BEFORE STARTING DIALYSIS

People with kidney failure who have not yet started dialysis should follow normal healthy eating guidelines. This includes continuing to eat foods that contain protein even after the level of urea in their blood has started to rise.

If people with kidney failure restrict their intake of dietary protein, their urea level will not rise so rapidly. For this reason, it has been suggested that reducing the amount of protein in the diet might delay the need for dialysis. Such use of protein restriction is controversial, since lower levels of urea in the blood may indicate that patients are becoming malnourished – i.e. they do not receive enough protein to maintain their flesh weight (see page 20). However, in some countries (e.g. Italy) doctors still recommend reducing protein intake, largely by use of a vegetarian diet.

When the time for dialysis draws closer, some people do not feel as hungry as they used to – and some foods, particularly meat products, may taste 'funny'. Special dietary supplements may help such patients to maintain adequate protein, energy and vitamin intakes. A dietitian will be able to provide advice about these supplements.

DIET DURING DIALYSIS

Several aspects of diet and nutrition are very important for patients on dialysis. All kidney patients are at an increased risk of developing malnutrition (see below).

It may also be necessary to pay special attention to a dialysis patient's intake of phosphate, calcium, potassium, salt, fluid and vitamins (see pages 106–7). In some cases, there may also be other specific individual dietary recommendations (see page 107).

GAINING WEIGHT AND KIDNEY FAILURE

Even though weight loss is a problem that causes particular concern in kidney failure (see page 105), weight gain (obesity) can be also be an issue.

Obesity can actually contribute to the development of kidney failure. This is largely because being overweight makes a person much more likely to develop diabetes mellitus, one of the major causes of kidney failure.

Reversing obesity (losing weight by dieting) will not cure kidney failure. Nevertheless, the other health advantages, such as reducing blood pressure and strain on the heart, are well worth achieving. At the very least, patients on the transplant waiting list are more likely to cope physically with a transplant operation if they are a healthy weight and do not have raised blood pressure.

Obesity can cause practical problems for people on dialysis. Overweight people with fat arms can have particular problems with access for haemodialysis. Their veins can be difficult to reach, or weak, and therefore difficult to make a fistula from (see pages 70–1). It can be difficult to put a PD catheter into someone who has a very fat abdomen. Very obese patients will be too unfit to be offered a transplant.

If obesity is a problem, healthy eating guidelines may

help. Overweight patients should ask to be referred to a dietitian for advice.

LOSING WEIGHT AND KIDNEY FAILURE

Some kidney patients find they lose a lot of weight and become very thin. This is usually because they are not eating enough (especially foods providing protein and energy). Loss of appetite is often one of the first things people notice when their kidneys stop working properly. Such patients rapidly become malnourished.

Malnutrition is the most important, and most dangerous, nutritional problem that can develop in patients on either type of dialysis. So, to prevent malnutrition, some patients on dialysis will be asked to increase their food intake – especially their intake of protein.

Doctors are not entirely sure why kidney patients have an increased risk of malnutrition, and why they need extra protein in their diet. A combination of causes seems most likely.

POOR APPETITE AND MALNUTRITION

The most important cause of malnutrition in kidney patients is probably the simplest one – poor appetite. This is one of the major symptoms of kidney failure, and is often the reason why people go to their family doctor in the first place.

When someone is pre-dialysis (or has a failing transplant), worsening of the appetite is one of the reasons why doctors start (or restart) dialysis. When a patient is on dialysis, a change – hopefully an improvement – in their appetite is often the most reliable guide to the effectiveness of the dialysis. It can tell more than any of the blood tests (including the 'key' test, the blood creatinine, see Chapter 2).

Dialysis usually restores a kidney patient's appetite to near normal, although few dialysis patients ever really have a 'good' appetite. Dialysis is just not good enough at getting rid of the toxins that suppress appetite. (Doctors do not even know which these toxins are.)

If there is under-dialysis (i.e. a patient is not receiving enough dialysis), loss of appetite is one of the first symptoms of kidney failure to return. An increase in the dialysis dose will then probably help to improve the patient's appetite. However, only a transplant will fully return a patient to a 'normal' appetite.

A build-up of toxins in the blood may not be the only reason for appetite problems in a kidney patient. Severe anaemia (see Chapter 5) may also suppress appetite.

Also, PD patients may have a poor appetite because of the dialysis fluid in their abdomen, which can make them feel bloated.

OTHER CAUSES OF WEIGHT LOSS

In addition to appetite problems, a number of other factors may contribute to the increased risk of weight loss in kidney patients on dialysis.

PD patients lose protein and amino acids (substances from which proteins are built up) into their bags of dialysis fluid. Haemodialysis patients also lose amino acids into their dialysis fluid. So kidney patients on both types of dialysis need extra protein in their diet to make up for these losses.

Poor control of blood acidity level (blood tends to be acidic in kidney failure) is another important factor. This is shown by low bicarbonate levels in the blood (see page 42). A research study carried out by Dr Stein showed that dialysis patients with higher bicarbonate levels (less acidic blood) were more likely to be alive and better nourished after the first year of dialysis.

Infections also increase a person's requirements for high-protein and high-energy foods, and infections tend to be more common in dialysis patients.

A further possible cause of malnutrition in kidney patients may be that some patients are not eating enough because of dietary restrictions imposed by their doctor or dietitian. Fortunately, such over-zealous dietary restrictions are now going out of fashion.

Loss of weight tends to be more common in haemodialysis than PD patients. PD patients have an extra source of calories – the sugar contained in PD fluid. Some of this is absorbed by the patient, providing the equivalent of approximately 300–500 calories a day – similar to eating between one and two Mars Bars. Haemodialysis patients don't have this extra energy source and may need additional dietary advice and supplements.

PROTEIN/ENERGY SUPPLEMENTS

Protein and/or energy supplements can be helpful if a kidney patient is not eating enough. These supplements are really very good and supply varying amounts of protein and energy depending on what is needed. They are available on prescription, and hospital dietitians can ask their patients' GPs to prescribe them.

PHOSPHATE AND CALCIUM

Phosphate and calcium are two minerals that affect the health of the bones. When a person has kidney failure, the calcium level in their body tends to be too low, and their phosphate level too high. This puts them at risk of bone problems, due to a condition called renal bone disease (see Chapter 6).

Treatment for kidney patients therefore aims to raise blood calcium levels and also to lower blood phosphate levels. Both these aims can often be achieved by:

- reducing the phosphate content of your diet;

- adequate dialysis if this has been started; and

- using a phosphate binder (calcium carbonate, e.g. Calcichew) taken as tablets with meals.

A low-phosphate diet is not as straightforward as it sounds. It is very difficult to cut down phosphate intake without also lowering protein intake.

Patients who need to adjust their diet to reduce their blood phosphate level will be given specific advice by their dietitian. This will probably include asking them to be careful about eating dairy produce, offal and shellfish – as these all contain particularly high amounts of phosphate. The dietitian may also give advice about the distribution and timing of phosphate-binding tablets.

In general, patients only need to worry about the amount of phosphate in their diet if their doctor or dietitian specifically tells them they have a problem.

POTASSIUM

Potassium is another very important mineral in the human body. The kidneys normally regulate potassium level without any difficulty, but in kidney failure this control is lost. Potassium levels may then be either too high or too low (see Chapter 7, page 41).

The main problem with potassium is that if it rises to a very high (or falls to a very low) level in the blood, it becomes dangerous to the heart, which can stop beating.

Potassium is one of the substances that is measured when dialysis patients have blood tests. Any patient who regularly has high blood potassium levels will get to know their dietitian very well. The dietitian will try to find out if the person is eating anything that might be causing a high level of potassium in the blood.

Many foods contain potassium, but some have more than others. Kidney patients whose blood potassium levels are high or rising will normally be asked to restrict their intake of high-potassium foods. This will involve avoiding some (rather nice) foods, such as chocolate and crisps, and moderating their intake of other potassium-containing foods, such as bananas, oranges and mushrooms. If this dietary restriction does not work, the dietitian may recommend an increase in dialysis dose, usually an increase in the number of hours per haemodialysis session.

Patients on more frequent or continuous forms of dialysis such as daily home haemodialysis, night-time haemodialysis, or PD rarely need to restrict their potassium intake, and in fact may sometimes need to increase it.

This is because more frequent dialysis generally clears potassium from the blood very effectively. Hospital or satellite-based haemodialysis, on the other hand, is an intermittent process. So, in the intervals between dialysis, the blood potassium may begin to rise. These patients may therefore need dietary advice on potassium intake.

Unless their doctor or dietitian tells them otherwise, kidney patients can assume that they do not have a problem with their blood potassium.

WHAT ABOUT SALT AND FLUID?

Salt and fluid advice are often given together. A salty diet may make patients thirsty, and make life very uncomfortable if a fluid restriction is necessary.

Salt restriction usually involves the following:

- using little or no salt in cooking and at the table;

- decreasing the intake of high-salt foods, which are mainly convenience and processed foods.

Hospital or satellite-based haemodialysis patients often have greater restrictions on fluid intake as their dialysis is intermittent and fluid can build up in between sessions. They therefore need to be extra careful about the amount of salt they eat.

Fluid advice for individual kidney patients is based on a combination of their urine output (if they still pass urine) and the amount of water removed by dialysis. Generally speaking, the more urine patients pass, the more fluid they can drink. A common generalisation is that dialysis patients can drink 500 ml of fluid every day plus the

equivalent of any urine they have passed plus any fluid lost by dialysis on the previous day. For many patients, this works out to be about 1 litre for haemodialysis patients and 1.5 litres for PD patients.

VITAMIN SUPPLEMENTS

There are different opinions about the value of vitamin supplements for people who have kidney failure.

Most doctors and dietitians agree that the so-called fat-soluble vitamins (i.e. vitamins A, D, E and K) are rarely a problem and don't need supplementing. Supplements of fat-soluble vitamins may even cause problems, as excessive amounts accumulate in the body. One fat-soluble vitamin – vitamin A (found in large amounts in cod and halibut liver oil capsules) – is known to be toxic and can cause problems if taken to excess.

It is known that the so-called water-soluble vitamins (i.e. vitamins B and C) are lost in both types of dialysis. It is therefore possible that there may be deficiencies if patients reduce their intake of certain foods, either voluntarily or because of potassium restrictions. A case can therefore be made for supplementing these vitamins. But should everyone take supplements, just to make sure, bearing in mind the large number of tablets most kidney patients are taking anyway? Different units adopt different policies.

INDIVIDUAL DIETARY RECOMMENDATIONS

All people with kidney failure are advised, as far as possible, to follow 'healthy eating guidelines' (i.e. to eat a high-fibre, moderate-fat and low-salt diet). But in some cases, specific individual priorities will over-ride these guidelines.

The most common example of going against the usual guidelines is if someone is losing a lot of weight and needs to boost their intake of calories with fat. In this situation, malnutrition is a more serious and immediate danger than any possible future increased risk of heart disease from a high-fat diet. Hence the reason for the 'unhealthy' compromise on fat intake.

DIET AFTER A TRANSPLANT

A common question after someone has had a kidney transplant is, 'Do I still need to follow a special diet?' The simple answer is, 'No'. If a kidney is functioning well, then there is no need to be on a special diet. If the transplant starts to fail, the situation may be different.

Transplant patients, being immuno-suppressed and at greater risk than other people of picking up infections, should be given information about food hygiene. In addition, they will be advised to follow normal healthy eating guidelines. This is particularly important because of two problems associated with a transplant. Both these problems – excessive weight gain (usually a side effect of taking steroid drugs, such as prednisolone) and high cholesterol levels – increase the risk of heart disease. Healthy eating habits may help reduce the risk.

TAKING CONTROL OF WHAT YOU EAT

Diet is an area where you really can take some control over your lifestyle and feel you are doing something to improve your own situation. Having kidney failure does not mean you have to stop enjoying your food. What it does mean is that you need to understand what you are eating, and learn which foods you can eat as much of as you like; which foods you should have once in a while (as a treat) and which foods you really should consider cutting out altogether. It is important though that, while you follow your doctor and dietitian's advice, you do not become so obsessed with watching the relative values of everything you eat that meals become a chore for you. The Further Reading list on page 159 lists some books that will help you find the right balance.

KEY FACTS

1 Advice about what you should eat will vary according to the stage of kidney failure and the type of treatment you are receiving.

2 'Healthy eating guidelines' – for high-fibre, moderate-fat and low-salt diet – are generally recommended whether you are waiting for dialysis, are on dialysis or have a transplant.

3 It is difficult to measure someone's nutritional state. The blood albumin level is often used, but is not very reliable. A low level may be a sign of malnutrition in some cases.

4 You should only alter your diet when your kidney doctor or dietitian advises you to.

5 Weight gain can lead to practical problems if you need dialysis. It may also make you too unfit for a transplant operation.

6 Weight loss and malnutrition are the major problems for many patients on dialysis. So, for these patients, eating a lot of high-protein food may be recommended.

7 If you are on frequent or continuous dialysis treatments such as PD or daily home haemodialysis, it is unlikely you will need to reduce your potassium intake. But you may need to restrict it if you are on hospital or satellite-based haemodialysis three times a week.

8 Eating a lot of salt or salty foods will make you thirsty. You may need to restrict your salt intake, particularly if fluid is restricted.

9 If you have had a transplant, you are unlikely to have any dietary restrictions. But you should try to follow standard healthy eating guidelines.

15 LIVING WITH KIDNEY FAILURE

This chapter looks at the reasons why people with kidney failure may feel differently from people with healthy kidneys. It also suggests ways of coping with the psychological problems you may experience as you adapt to life with kidney failure.

INTRODUCTION

A diagnosis of kidney failure has a massive impact. It will affect the whole of your life, not just your physical condition. Once you know you have kidney failure, you will have to make changes to the way you live. You are also likely to find the illness affects the way you feel about yourself, and your priorities in life.

BODY AND MIND

Everyone's psychological and emotional well-being has a major impact on their physical well-being. The way you feel will influence the way you behave.

The way kidney patients behave has a direct effect on their physical condition. They may become less careful about their diet, forget to take their tablets, or abandon fluid restrictions – all of which put additional strain on an already poorly body.

PSYCHOLOGICAL NEEDS

Psychology is about behaviour: why people behave the way they do, and how they can change the way they behave. It is about how people feel about themselves,

their situation, the people who are part of their lives. Everybody has psychological needs – not just people who happen to have kidney failure. However old or ill we might be, we all need to be heard, understood and valued. Illness can make this more difficult. People who are unwell may find it hard to express their fears and anxieties, or feel in control of the situation.

STRESSES ON PEOPLE WITH KIDNEY FAILURE

Any long-term or life-threatening illness, can be extremely stressful. Any change – even a pleasant change like getting married – is stressful. When changes are 'negative', however, stress will be greatly increased.

The treatment of kidney failure means you can't avoid changes in lifestyle. People have to adapt their usual routine. They may have to make changes to their eating and drinking habits. They may not have sufficient energy to continue working or to pursue hobbies or interests.

Some of the stresses that commonly affect people with kidney failure are:

- having to make decisions about things they have never even thought about before;

- taking in strange information, to enable them to understand a complex medical subject;

- learning about themselves and the ways they cope with things;

- needing to ask for support to manage their treatment;

- seeing themselves as a complete person, not just as a disease or condition;

- learning to live differently for the rest of their life; and

- worrying about the future.

Changes to the expected progression of life may also cause stress. For example, it may be difficult for a young person to leave home, either because they have kidney failure, or because they feel they should look after a parent with kidney failure. Sometimes people have to cope with unpleasant reactions from their employers and work colleagues. Later in life, retirement may come early and be totally unwelcome.

Other members of the family also have to make adjustments. Kidney failure has an impact on their lives too. The normal pattern of life is disrupted and relationships have to be redefined.

THE DIAGNOSIS

For some people, the diagnosis of kidney failure comes completely out of the blue. This can be extremely difficult to cope with. Even when kidney failure was already suspected, knowing it is definite can cause difficulties. The way that the diagnosis is given, and the quality of support offered immediately afterwards, can make a big difference to a person's future well-being.

INITIAL REACTIONS

Following a diagnosis of kidney failure (or any other serious long-term illness), people typically go through the following stages:

1. Shock. At first, patients (and sometimes also family members and friends) go into a state of shock, feeling stunned, bewildered or strangely detached – as though they are observing life rather than being part of it. This shock can last a short while or may continue for weeks.

2. Grief. Then people begin to react to the news, often with feelings of loss, grief, helplessness and despair. They may feel overwhelmed by reality, and find it difficult to think clearly or plan effectively.

3. Denial. One very common reaction to serious illness is to deny the existence of the disease or its implications. But the problem does not go away, the symptoms get worse, and there are reminders from other people that the illness exists.

4. Acceptance. Gradually, people come to accept reality a little at a time, and begin to make progress towards adapting successfully to their condition.

LONGER-TERM PROBLEMS

Patients with kidney failure often experience longer-term psychological problems too. Some of these are described below:

1. Lack of co-operation with the medical team. Various terms have been used by doctors for 'not doing as you are told'. Until a few years ago, you may have heard the term 'non-compliance' or even 'non-adherence'. Now you are more likely to hear your health professionals using terms such as 'lack of concordance' in relation to an agreed programme of treatment and self-help measures. The term 'concordance' signifies mutual decision making between patient and health professionals. Reasons why patients may find it difficult to keep to the decisions about treatment and lifestyle that have been mutually agreed in this way include:

- they believe that the treatment is not effective, and there is no obvious benefit from it;

- they do not know what effect the treatment is supposed to have, or why it is important to continue with it; and

- the side effects of the treatment are unpleasant.

Almost a third of all patients will have at least one period when they find it difficult to follow the guidance set out by their doctors and nurses – after all, no one likes being told what to do.

You need to be aware, however, that if you don't follow your agreed treatment regime, you can end up very ill indeed. It is much better to learn how to manage your kidney failure by exploring with your doctor or nurse which areas allow you some flexibility, at the same time as being absolutely certain which are the situations where choosing not to follow your treatment plan can be life-threatening. Do talk to your renal unit team. If you understand why you should (or should not) be doing something, you will feel much more motivated about it. Many problems of this nature can be solved by better communication between doctors or nurses and their patients.

2. Anxiety. As well as the anxieties felt by most people at some time in their lives, kidney patients have additional anxieties relating to their condition and its treatment. Some possible problem areas include:

- relationships (e.g. 'We can't share the same interests any more'; 'We've both changed so much');

- quality of life (e.g. 'I miss walking the dog'; 'I'd planned to go abroad');

- employment (e.g. 'I've taken too much time off work');

- practical management (e.g. 'How can I do my dialysis myself when I feel so ill?'); and

- understanding (e.g. 'I can't understand all the medical words').

3. Body image. Not all people with kidney failure have problems with their changed body image, but some do. They may see their fistula or PD catheter as a defect in their body. They feel horribly scarred and find it really hard to look at themselves.

The perceptions of patients and medical staff can differ widely here. When doctors and nurses talk about a 'really good fistula', they are talking about the ease of access, the rate of blood flow, and the strength of the blood vessels. What the patient experiences is a forearm with a continuous buzzing sensation, and a disfiguring swelling where it used to be smooth and flat. Some patients cannot see their fistula as a 'good' thing at all.

4. Awareness of early death. People with kidney failure know that without treatment they would die. Having to live with this sort of knowledge puts a very different perspective on life's priorities.

5. Dependency and self-confidence. Kidney patients are very dependent – on hospital doctors and nurses, and on their partners, relatives and friends. People with kidney failure have to deal with the fact that their life depends on a machine, on PD bags, or on someone else's kidney. This necessary dependency can undermine a person's confidence in coping with both kidney and non-kidney issues.

If issues relating to dependency and self-confidence are not dealt with, they may cause conflict between kidney patients and hospital staff or carers.

6. Sense of loss. A person's kidneys have been a part of them since birth. A healthy person will take their kidneys (and every other organ) for granted, never having to think about them. So the failure of this essential body part is likely to give rise to a kind of grieving.

7. Depression. Most people get depressed at some stage in their lives. Periods of depression may be useful, in that they enable people to withdraw from the world for a while, and resolve certain issues. People with kidney failure are no exception. There are times when they feel low, and to do anything at all requires a huge effort; times when they should allow themselves to feel sorry for themselves; and times to cry.

8. Changes to treatment. One of the many difficult things about kidney failure is that the treatment changes over time. For example, patients may change from PD to haemodialysis, or vice versa, or they may receive a transplant, or resume dialysis after a transplant fails.

9. Ageing and bereavement. It is not only a patient's treatment that changes. Everyone changes to some extent as they get older. Tasks that seem easy when someone is young may become more troublesome as the years go by. Coping with kidney failure may become more difficult.

Everyone (perhaps those in perfect health most of all) finds that, as they get older, more and more of their friends will die. This can be a particular problem for older patients in the kidney unit. In addition, if you attend the same unit for a long time, you may see many staff changes. Just as you are building up a rapport with one dialysis nurse, they move to a new job or retire. This can become a strong and supportive relationship and the better it is the more difficult you may find it to adjust to their not being around.

10. Sexual activity. Sexual problems are very common among people with kidney failure and can put strain on a relationship. Concerns about sexual ability vary from person to person. There may be a loss of sex drive, especially in men. For many young men, the most distressing aspect of kidney failure is their inability to get or maintain a normal erection. Women may worry about whether they can get pregnant, or have a healthy baby. (See *Chapter 16* for more information about sexual problems and fertility.)

11. Conflicting advice. People with kidney failure receive information from lots of different people. The people who pass on this information have themselves already interpreted it according to their own backgrounds and beliefs. So, what a patient hears may not always be totally true. The advice from one source may conflict directly with advice from another. It is not surprising that kidney patients are sometimes confused by what they are told.

12. Poor concentration. Patients sometimes worry that kidney failure may be affecting their brain. They may find that they sometimes cannot concentrate as well, or think as clearly, as they used to before their kidneys failed. These problems may last from a few minutes to several days at a time. However, for most people with kidney failure, most of the time, the ability to concentrate and think clearly is as good as it ever was. When there are problems, efficient dialysis will often help a patient to think straight.

FACTORS AFFECTING THE ABILITY TO COPE

Some people cope more easily than others with the psychological and emotional aspects of kidney failure. Research indicates that an individual's ability to cope with illness is influenced by a range of factors:

1. Illness-related factors. The first group of factors relates to the illness itself:

- Some people are more afraid than others of the possible consequences of kidney failure. Fears of disability, disfigurement, pain or early death may need to be addressed. The more they feel threatened by their illness, the harder they will find it to cope.

- Kidney failure often occurs together with other conditions, such as diabetes, anaemia (see *Chapter 5*) and renal bone disease (see *Chapter 6*). These conditions cause their own symptoms, giving kidney patients even more things to worry about.

- Some people have to cope with unpleasant side effects from the tablets they must take (particularly if they have had a transplant, see *Chapter 13*).

- The treatment of kidney failure involves major time commitments, which can interfere with finding or holding down a job. Lack of secure employment can be an additional strain.

- Kidney failure requires patients and their families to make changes in their lifestyle. These changes may put pressure on relationships and increase stress.

- Many people with a chronic illness, such as kidney failure, feel self-conscious about their disease and want to hide it from others. This can cause stress and make it harder to cope.

2. Age. The age at which a person develops kidney failure is likely to influence the way they will cope:

- Children may not understand the long-term implications of the condition.

- Adolescents need to be liked and accepted by their peers. Because of this, some may neglect their medical care to avoid appearing different from their friends.

- Young adults with kidney failure may feel they no longer have the chance to develop their lives in the direction they planned – to get married, to have children, or to enter a particular career. Such feelings may cause anger and resentment.

- Middle-aged patients may have problems adjusting to the disruption of an established lifestyle. They may find themselves unable to finish tasks they have started, such as building up a business.

- Older patients may resent not being able to enjoy their retirement.

3. Personality. Aspects of a person's personality can affect their ability to cope with kidney failure:

- People who cope well with long-term health problems tend to have hardy or resilient personalities which allow them to see good in difficult situations. They are able to balance hope against despair and to find purpose in life whatever happens. They maintain their self-esteem and resist feeling helpless and hopeless.

- Kidney failure often means that patients must take on a dependent and passive role, for a while at least. Some people find this especially difficult since it is so different from the independent role they have developed over the years.

4. Social and cultural factors. A person's ability to cope with illness is also affected by their background:

- People from different social, cultural and religious backgrounds will have different ways of dealing with situations. Problems may arise if doctors and nurses fail to take this into account.

- People's beliefs about health come from a number of sources, including the media, advertising, other patients' experiences and their friends. These beliefs may be incorrect or only half true.

Sometimes, misconceptions can add to the difficulties of adjusting to kidney failure. For instance, people who believe that nothing is seriously wrong unless they are in pain are not likely to seek help for a condition that has no obvious symptoms, such as high blood pressure.

5. Support. The amount and quality of support available to patients are further influences on how well they cope with kidney failure:

- People who live alone, away from their family and with few friends, tend to adjust poorly to long-term diseases. Other forms of support are particularly important for these people.

- For many people with kidney failure, the immediate family is the main source of psychological support. For others, this role is taken by one or more close friends. Such support is usually a big help to the person. However, it is also true that relatives and friends sometimes undermine effective coping by providing bad examples or poor advice.

- Hospitals do not always provide people with kidney failure with the support they need. Hospitals can be dull places for patients, and further depress their mood. Unfortunately, at present, not all renal units have a clinical psychologist. However, there is a general recognition of the need to provide patients with psychological support, and some nurses have had special training in counselling.

- For some people, lack of practical support at home may be a problem. Patients may have difficulty getting round the house or doing everyday tasks. Many lack equipment that could help them become more self-sufficient.

- Many support groups have been set up by and for people with kidney failure. These groups can provide emotional and sometimes financial support, as well as information. (See the 'Useful Addresses' section on *page 160*.)

COPING STRATEGIES

People with kidney failure use different strategies to help them cope with this long-term illness. Many kidney patients find the following strategies helpful:

1. Denial. In the early stages, it can be very useful to deny the situation or not to take it seriously. This helps people escape from the feeling of being overwhelmed by the disease. It also allows time to organise other, better ways of dealing with the situation. The belief that a person with kidney failure is still the same as everyone else is a very important element in psychological well-being.

2. Information seeking. People often find it helpful to seek information about their disease and its treatment. Becoming expert in a subject may give you a sense of control over it. It is particularly important that you feel able to ask your doctor or nurse questions, and that you ask them to explain anything they have told you in words that are easy for you to understand. There is also a great deal of other information available, from books and websites. The quality of this information does vary considerably, but all the sources listed on pages 159–164 have been looked at by the authors and have been found to be reliable.

3. Disease management. Many patients gain a sense of control over their disease by becoming involved in its management – including being responsible for tablet taking and perhaps doing their own dialysis at home. Some people find it helpful to keep their own records (for example, of their blood pressure, creatinine, eGFR, Hb, potassium and phosphate levels). It is a good idea to keep these in a file along with copies of all clinic letters and discharge summaries; notes of appointments at the renal clinic (dated, and with a record of who was seen and what decisions were made); details and dates of any operations or other procedures undergone, together with the names of the surgeon, anaesthetist and any other health professionals involved.

4. Goal setting. A very useful coping strategy for many people is to set themselves appropriate goals. These might include, for example, exercising or going out, and trying to maintain regular routines.

5. Thinking positively. One of the problems can often be that bad news travels better than good. Join your local kidney patients' association and talk to people who are managing to maintain a good quality of life on dialysis or with a transplant. What can you learn about coping from them? Kidney failure may change your life, but it doesn't need to destroy it.

6. Prioritising different activities. Some people with kidney failure, find it can be helpful in the long term to reduce the importance of some of their current activities, such as social drinking or playing contact sports. Maintaining some of the things you did before you had kidney failure is also important. Work, education and travel may have been a significant part of life, and with planning, are perfectly possible to continue.

WORKING

Employers are usually very accommodating towards people with kidney failure. Keeping them informed of changes to your treatment and the frequency of hospital visits help with their understanding of your requirements. People who have their dialysis at home often don't have a problem fitting work into their life. Home dialysis (either PD or haemodialysis) is flexible and, if dialysis is done overnight (by APD for example), it may interfere

very little with work schedules. Hospital or satellite-based haemodialysis may be more difficult to fit into a job, however, the renal unit may be able to offer a 'dialysis slot' that enables work to continue.

People who have a successful kidney transplant are usually able to work. However, in the early days after the operation, visits to the hospital can be much more frequent, especially if the patient was on a home-based treatment before the transplant. It's important to keep employers informed so they are prepared for possible disruptions to work patterns.

TRAVEL AND HOLIDAYS

One of the ways in which kidney patients can enjoy full and productive lives is by taking a holiday or business trip. For most people with kidney failure, travel to most parts of the world is perfectly possible, however planning is essential. Last-minute bookings are not a realistic option. There is plenty of help available with the planning process, beginning with your renal unit. Travel can give close family members a welcome break too.

Staff at the renal unit can help you decide if you are ready to travel. They can advise you on suitable destinations according to the treatment you are on. They can help you make appointments in other renal units so you can be monitored or treated while travelling.

Before planning anything, talk to your renal unit. Anyone with a pre-existing medical condition will need a letter from a doctor confirming that they are fit to travel in order to get travel insurance. This includes transplant patients. For more information about travel and holidays visit the websites recommended in the back of this book or contact the National Kidney Federation (*see page 163*). Your doctor or renal care team can also provide you with information about any immunisations required.

Short trips away are possible for patients on dialysis. Those on haemodialysis can plan a short trip away between dialysis sessions – especially on the two-day gap (e.g. Saturday and Sunday).

Peritoneal dialysis patients, on the other hand, are free to travel anytime as supplies can be taken along in the car. For longer trips away, PD supplies can be delivered to most parts of the world and will be waiting for you when you arrive at your destination. It's even possible to have PD on a cruise, or while camping.

Haemodialysis patients wishing to take a longer break away from home will need to organise dialysis in a unit near to their destination. Holiday dialysis centres are available in many parts of the world but need to be booked in advance.

KEY FACTS

1 Kidney failure has a major impact on the whole of a patient's life.

2 Psychology is about behaviour and beliefs.

3 People with kidney failure have to cope with extra stresses.

4 Kidney failure and its treatment will affect the lives of those who are closest to you, as well as your own.

5 People diagnosed with kidney failure (in common with people affected by many other serious diseases or trauma) usually go through shock, grief and denial before acceptance.

6 Deciding not to follow the treatment guidelines your doctor has given you is referred to as a 'lack of concordance'. Almost a third of patients choose not to follow an agreed treatment regime at some time or another.

7 Failing to follow your treatment regime can be very dangerous and even cause death – so it is vital you ask your doctor to talk through any aspect of your treatment programme you don't feel happy with or find difficult.

8 Other long-term problems may include anxiety, problems with body image, loss of self-confidence, depression, adapting to changes, and a loss of interest in sex.

9 Kidney failure can sometimes affect a person's ability to concentrate and think clearly. Efficient dialysis helps most people.

10 Many factors affect a person's ability to cope with kidney failure, but there are various coping strategies that different people find useful.

11 Some people prefer not to think about the situation, or refuse to take it seriously (denial). Others may adopt a structured approach, managing their own illness as far as possible, doing their dialysis at home, prioritising different activities or goal setting. It is important you follow the approach that works best for you.

12 Maintaining some of the things you did before you had kidney failure is important. It is perfectly possible to continue work, education and travel but they may require advance planning.

16 SEXUAL PROBLEMS AND PREGNANCY

This chapter describes the problems commonly experienced by men and women with kidney failure. It examines the causes of these problems, and makes some suggestions for what can be done about them.

INTRODUCTION

Although some kidney patients never have sexual problems, many others do. Sometimes, sexual problems start quite early in kidney failure, before dialysis is needed. Patients may then experience an improvement in their sex lives when they start dialysis, although some notice no difference. Other patients with kidney failure develop sexual problems only after they start dialysis (either PD or haemodialysis). A kidney transplant often improves a person's sex life, but problems may continue.

INVESTIGATING SEXUAL PROBLEMS

In the past, many health professionals working with kidney patients have tended to avoid getting involved with their patients' sexual problems. Patients, doctors and nurses have often been embarrassed to discuss the subject. Even now, despite the more general interest in and openness about sexual matters, people with kidney failure may still find that they have to raise the subject first.

As with other aspects of kidney failure, it is not usually a case of just one straightforward problem that can be easily corrected. Often there are several issues to look at, and patience is required. Nevertheless, treatment is usually successful, provided both partners are keen to have a sex life and are willing to accept help.

ERECTILE DYSFUNCTION (IMPOTENCE)

Men with kidney failure have a variety of sexual problems. These include having sex less often, loss of interest in sex (sometimes called loss of libido), and being unable to ejaculate ('come'). However, the most common sexual problem – and often the most worrying one for a man – is difficulty in getting or keeping a hard penis. This was generally known as 'impotence' but you may well find your doctor uses the term 'erectile dysfunction' or 'ED' instead.

What normally happens first in men with kidney failure is that they become less able to keep an erection for as long as usual, although they are still able to ejaculate. Eventually, many kidney patients lose the ability to get a hard penis at all. Obviously, this can lead to frustration, particularly if the sex drive is unchanged. The situation can be even more upsetting if the man's partner interprets the problem as a loss of interest in her personally.

WHAT CAUSES ERECTILE DYSFUNCTION?

Erectile dysfunction has many possible causes. In most men with kidney failure, sexual problems do not have just one cause, but are usually due to a combination of:

1. Poor blood supply. In order to make the penis hard, extra blood enters the penis and is then prevented from leaving it. Many kidney patients have narrowed blood vessels all over their body, including those vessels that supply the penis. This reduces the blood supply to the penis, and makes it difficult to get an erection. It is not just kidney patients who have this problem. It also occurs as part of the natural ageing process and is more common in older men as well as in men with diabetes.

2. Leaky blood vessels. To keep the penis hard, the extra blood that has entered the penis must stay inside it. In men with kidney failure, the extra blood sometimes leaks back out of the penis, and so the erection is lost.

3. Hormonal disturbances. Hormones are chemical messengers that control many body functions. They are carried around the body in the blood. Some hormones are specifically designed to control sexual urges. The levels of these sex hormones can be either higher or lower than normal in people with kidney failure. In particular, the testicles may produce less of the male sex hormone, testosterone.

4. Nerve damage. The nerves that supply the penis are also involved in getting an erection. When someone has kidney failure, nerve damage may prevent the nerves from working properly.

5. Tablets. Most tablets do not cause erectile dysfunction on their own. However, a few drugs can contribute to sexual problems. The biggest culprits are the blood pressure tablets called beta-blockers, such as atenolol, propranolol, metoprolol and bisoprolol.

6. Tiredness. Tiredness can affect sexual performance. Tiredness in a kidney patient may be caused by anaemia

(see *Chapter 5*), by under-dialysis (see *page 14*), or by other medical problems, such as heart problems.

7. Psychological problems. When a kidney patient starts dialysis, there are many stresses to deal with (see *Chapter 15*). Not surprisingly, some patients feel quite depressed. If so, they may not feel like having sex.

8. Relationship difficulties. The illness of one partner naturally causes stresses in a relationship. For instance, household jobs such as decorating or mowing the lawn, which used to be done by the patient, may now have to be done by the partner. This can lead to arguments or resentment on either side of the relationship.

The normal erection process

Signals from nerves supplying the genitals cause the main artery of the penis (a) to widen. Extra blood enters the spongy areas of the penis (b) making them swell. The swelling squeezes the veins that carry blood from the penis (c), trapping blood in the penis and making it swell even more

HOW IS ERECTILE DYSFUNCTION INVESTIGATED?

The first and most important step is for the subject to be raised. There is often a lot of unnecessary suffering due either to denial of the problem or to fear of embarrassment. Some kidney doctors and nurses have no experience of treating sexual problems in people with kidney failure, or are embarrassed themselves. If this is the case, patients should ask to see an expert in sexual problems. Sadly, few kidney units have access to such an expert at present.

Once the problem of erectile dysfunction has been recognised, the following should take place:

1. A general health check. This will include an assessment of the distance a person can walk on level ground without having to stop, which is a useful guide to general health.

2. Physical examination. This will include an examination of the genitals. The doctor will also feel for a pulse at various points in the legs. If the pulses are weak, this means that the blood vessels in the legs have narrowed, reducing the blood supply. There will then usually also be narrowing of the blood vessels supplying the penis, reducing its blood supply.

3. Blood tests. In addition to the usual blood tests, there will be tests to measure the blood levels of various hormones. These include testosterone, and also luteinising hormone (LH), follicle-stimulating hormone (FSH) and prolactin. LH and FSH are hormones that regulate the testicles. Prolactin's usual role is to produce milk in females, but it is often present in larger than normal amounts in male dialysis patients with erectile dysfunction.

4. Review of medication. The doctor should review the various tablets that the person is taking. Some types of tablet may contribute to sexual difficulties. Alternative medication is sometimes available.

5. Investigation of psycho-sexual problems. The doctor will ask the patient to consider whether psychological or relationship difficulties may be contributing to the physical problem of erectile dysfunction.

HOW IS ERECTILE DYSFUNCTION TREATED?

The doctor will begin by looking at any more general problems that may be contributing to erectile dysfunction. These may include:

- treating anaemia (see *Chapter 5*);
- increasing the amount of dialysis; and
- changing the patient's tablets.

More specific physical treatments for erectile dysfunction will then be considered. These may include:

- tablets (Viagra, Levitra, Cialis);
- hormone treatment;
- use of a vacuum device;
- penile injection therapy;
- penile insertion therapy (putting a drug down the penis); and
- penile implants.

In addition to the various physical treatment options (see *below* for more details), patients may be recommended to seek help for emotional problems relating to erectile dysfunction (see *page 122*).

Men who are on dialysis or have a kidney transplant can have treatment for erectile dysfunction free of charge on the NHS. People who are not getting treatment for kidney failure (i.e. dialysis or a transplant) may not be able to get free treatment for erection difficulties. However, if the doctor thinks the problems caused by erectile dysfunction are causing a lot of distress, treatment might be free.

TABLETS (VIAGRA, LEVITRA AND CIALIS)

Viagra (sildenafil) is the best known tablet for treating erectile dysfunction. It has had a lot of publicity since it first became available in America in April 1998. It works by opening up the blood vessels in the penis. This causes the man to have an erection.

An early trial of Viagra in kidney patients with erectile dysfunction who also had diabetes showed that the drug worked well in about half of them. However, they did get some side effects from the drug. These were occasional headaches, indigestion and muscle aches. People who have a condition called angina and use GTN (a spray which relieves the pain), and people who have very low blood pressure, should not take Viagra.

During the past few years, Viagra has become the first choice of treatment for kidney patients with erection problems. It works well in around 75% of the dialysis and transplant patients (diabetic or not) who take it. Many patients even say it lasts longer than usual – it can still be effective 'the morning after'!

Two other drugs, Levitra (vardenafil) and Cialis (tadalafil) have similar effects. Some doctors think these two drugs may not be suitable for all people with kidney failure. However, other drugs are being developed all the time.

HORMONES

Most male dialysis patients with sexual problems have lowish testosterone levels. This deficiency can be treated by an injection of testosterone every 3–4 weeks, or by using testosterone replacement patches (such as the Andropatch). Although testosterone therapies replace the hormone that is lacking, they are not always very effective in treating impotence. This is probably because impotence in men with kidney failure is not usually due only to low testosterone levels.

Many other hormones are also often found to be at the wrong level, but correcting them rarely makes much difference to sexual difficulties. If the prolactin level is too high, a tablet such as cabergoline or bromocriptine may be given. However, these tablets are not always very successful at making erection problems better.

VACUUM DEVICES

Many kidney patients with erectile dysfunction require therapies which act directly on the penis, helping them to get and keep an erection. One of these is called vacuum tumescence therapy, which uses a mechanical device (such as the ErecAid) to produce a hard penis. Nearly three quarters of the male dialysis patients who use a vacuum device are able to have full penile erections.

To use the vacuum device, the man first inserts his penis into the clear plastic cylinder. He then holds the device against his body so that the chamber is closed with an air-tight seal. Using either a hand- or battery-operated pump, the man then withdraws air from the cylinder to form a vacuum. This causes the penis to enlarge in a way that is similar to a natural erection. However, to maintain the erection, the man must then push a tension ring (resembling an elastic band) from the outside of the cylinder onto the base of the penis. The seal of the vacuum is broken, and the cylinder and pump are removed. With the tension ring in place, the erection can be maintained for up to 30 minutes.

The erections may be longer lasting than natural ones, and do not usually disappear after an orgasm. The most common complaints are mild discomfort and 'timing difficulties' (such as pumping too rapidly with the hand-pump) when the device is first used. Occasionally, harmless, tiny reddish spots (called petechiae) may appear on the penis.

The main advantages of vacuum therapy are that it is safe and non-surgical, can be used as often as desired, and works well for most male dialysis patients. Its suppliers also claim that it may improve blood flow to the penis and result in occasional natural erections.

An ErecAid

1 The man's penis is inserted into the plastic cylinder of the ErecAid. The ErecAid is then held against the body to form an airtight seal

penis | plastic cylinder

tension ring | pump

2 The man uses the pump to withdraw air from the cylinder forming a vacuum. The penis enlarges in a similar way to a natural erection

air withdrawn using pump

vacuum created inside cylinder

3 The tension ring is slipped off the ErecAid onto the base of the penis to help maintain the erection, and the ErecAid is then removed

tension ring on base of penis

The disadvantages of vacuum therapy are that it involves a loss of spontaneity in lovemaking, it requires some skill to use, and it can cause mild bruising.

PENILE INJECTION THERAPY

Penile injection therapy is another non-surgical technique used to treat erectile dysfunction. The man injects medication (usually alprostadil) into the base of his penis. This causes the penis to become hard almost immediately. The erection then lasts for 1–2 hours.

The use of the injection is limited to not more than once a day and three times a week. Several clinic visits are usually needed to establish the dose of medication required. The treatment is available on the NHS.

Penile injections have the advantage of not involving surgery. They are also effective in many dialysis patients. The main problems with this technique are pain in the penis, and a condition called priapism, which is an unwanted erection that goes on too long. There may also be bleeding, bruising or scarring (fibrosis) at the injection site. Because of the risk of bleeding, patients on haemodialysis are advised not to have the injection on a dialysis day because of the heparin used during dialysis (see page 75). Another problem is that the penis may become mis-shaped. After a while, some patients get fed up with having these injections, but it is usually possible for them to change to another type of treatment.

PENILE INSERTION (TRANSURETHRAL) THERAPY

Patients who use this treatment have to pass urine beforehand. This makes insertion of the pellet easier (because of the lubrication), and it also helps to dissolve the pellet. Some patients who don't pass much urine may therefore have difficulty using this treatment.

Penile insertion therapy, such as MUSE (Medicated Urethral System for Erection), involves the patient slowly inserting an applicator into the end of his penis. A button on the applicator is then pressed to release a tiny pellet of medication (alprostadil). Once the pellet has been released, the applicator is removed and an erection develops over the next 10–30 minutes.

Penile insertion therapy has been shown to be successful in just over half the men treated in the general population. The most common side effects are penile discomfort or burning, and light-headedness. Female partners have occasionally reported vaginal burning or itching.

Penile insertion therapy is likely to have a slightly higher failure rate than vacuum devices and penile injections. Nevertheless it is a safe, well-tolerated treatment option.

PENILE IMPLANTS

The decision to have a penile implant should be made only after very careful consideration. This surgical treatment for erectile dysfunction is usually effective, but it does have disadvantages (see *below*).

The implant is inserted during an operation performed under a general anaesthetic. There are various different types available. It is usual to have a cylinder implanted in the penis, and connected by a tube to a pump in the scrotum. This pump is connected by another tube to a fluid-containing reservoir in the abdomen (tummy). Squeezing the pump with the fingers causes fluid to pass from the reservoir into the cylinder, so simulating an erection.

The main disadvantage is that the operation to insert the implant alters the penis permanently, ending all hope of natural erections. There is also a risk of infection, and a possibility that the implant will be rejected by the immune system (the body's defence system). Another problem is that an implant can be difficult to conceal.

EMOTIONAL PROBLEMS

Even though the treatments described above usually help to correct erection difficulties, they cannot by themselves restore a sexual relationship.

Sexual problems involve two people, and both partners need to work hard to sort them out. It is very common for people to experience changes in loving relationships after the development of kidney failure. Often, early in kidney disease, one partner becomes the 'carer' and the other adopts the 'sick role'. Later, the improved health of a patient on dialysis, and the desire to restore a sexual relationship, can create new stresses which may take time and patience from both partners to resolve.

Other hidden fears may also be present. For instance, some people may believe that kidney disease could be transferred during sex. This is not true.

Many kidney patients and their partners may want to have counselling, from either a psychologist or a sexual counsellor. This can be very effective, so if you feel it might be helpful in your case, do talk to your GP or renal unit doctor about whether you can be referred to a specialist counsellor.

SEXUAL PROBLEMS FOR WOMEN

Many women who have kidney failure do not have problems with having sex and have happy and fulfilled sex lives. However, there are some specific problems that female patients may experience:

1. Discomfort during sex. Some women do find that sex is sometimes painful. This may be due to a problem with a lack of lubrication (producing juices in the vagina). If this is the case, having more foreplay can help, although using a water-based lubricant (like KY jelly), which is available over the counter from chemists, may be the answer. Another cause of painful sex in women is an infection of the vagina (for example, thrush) or of the womb. If an infection is present, it can easily be treated with antibiotic or antifungal medication.

2. Reduced sex drive. People who need regular dialysis often feel very tired, especially following a session on the haemodialysis machine. However, there are many other reasons why sex drive may be lower than usual, and these include depression, anaemia or a change in roles between partners.

One of the most important things a woman with

kidney failure can do is to make sure her partner knows her feelings for him haven't changed. She can make a point of letting him know he is still valued. Planning something romantic on the days when the tiredness isn't so bad can work wonders.

It is also a good idea to discuss the problems of tiredness and reduced sex drive with the doctor when visiting the kidney unit. The various medications prescribed may make the situation worse for some women.

3. Body image. Some kidney patients have problems and worries with the way they look, especially those on dialysis, because of either the catheter or fistula. This often leads to feeling self-conscious, unattractive and no longer desirable. This in turn can lead to them avoiding sex with their partner. However, it is often only the patient (and not the partner) who feels this way. The truth is that a woman with kidney failure is still the same person with the same lovable characteristics she had before her kidneys failed.

It is very common for patients to lose confidence in themselves and not feel like making love any more. But this can lead either partner to blame themselves, and think that they are no longer attractive. The easiest and often most effective remedy in these situations is to talk to each other. If both partners can reassure each other, and express affection for each other, they will each be well on the way to regaining their confidence.

Many kidney units now have a counsellor who is specially trained to deal with problems such as this. If you are worried and would like professional help, ask your nurse or doctor if you can see a counsellor.

MENSTRUAL PERIODS AND FERTILITY

It is common for the menstrual periods to become irregular when women develop kidney failure. If a woman with kidney failure does not yet need dialysis, she will be less fertile (less likely to become pregnant, even if she is having regular sex) than other women are. However, she should use contraception, as pregnancy is still possible.

In dialysis patients, the periods often stop completely. This means that women on dialysis are not very likely to

RISK OF PROBLEMS DURING PREGNANCY FOR KIDNEY PATIENTS

	Creatinine less than 120 µmol/l (CKF Stage 1)	Creatinine of between 120 and 250 µmol/l (CKF Stage 2–3)	Creatinine of more than 250 µmol/l (CKF Stages 4–5)
Chance of problems occurring during pregnancy	25%	50%	85%
Chance of the baby being born small		30%	60%
Chance of the baby being born prematurely		55%	70%
Chance of a successful pregnancy	85–95%	60–90%	20–30%

become pregnant. However, again, women should not rely on this as a form of contraception. It is still possible to get pregnant even without having periods.

Treatment with an erythropoietin stimulating agent (ESA) has been shown to restore menstrual periods in about 50% of women on dialysis. This is thought to be due to two effects of EPO. It improves disturbed hormone levels, and it treats anaemia (see Chapter 5). Treatment with an ESA increases a woman's chance of becoming pregnant, so contraception should always be used to avoid an unwanted pregnancy.

PREGNANCY

Many women of child-bearing age who are on dialysis have irregular periods or no periods at all, yet it is still possible for them to become pregnant. However, the success of pregnancy varies widely, depending on the degree of kidney failure. The easiest and most reliable way to calculate the risk to both mother and baby is by estimating the level of kidney function, and this is most easily done by measuring the level of creatinine in the blood. The table on page 123 shows the percentage chance of problems occurring, depending on the level of creatinine in the patient's blood when she becomes pregnant. As you can see, women who have a creatinine level of less than 120 µmol/l (micromoles per litre of blood) have a much better chance of a trouble-free pregnancy and having a healthy baby.

If a woman does become pregnant when she already has even mild kidney failure, there is a risk, despite the success of the pregnancy, that her kidney failure will worsen. If you do have kidney failure, but are not yet getting treatment (dialysis or a transplant), it is worth taking this into consideration before trying for a baby. The table below shows the likelihood of kidney damage during pregnancy, depending on the level of creatinine in the patient's blood.

Following a transplant, most women find their periods start again as their hormone levels return to normal, and there is better clearance of the toxins from the body. Oestradiol is one of the hormones controlling a woman's periods, and this is usually restored to normal after a transplant, resulting in a return of normal ovulation (egg

RISKS TO KIDNEY FUNCTION DURING PREGNANCY

	Creatinine less than 120 µmol/l (CKF Stage 1)	Creatinine of between 170 and 220 µmol/l (CKF Stage 2–3)	Creatinine of more than 220 µmol/l (CKF Stages 4–5)
Chance of losing kidney function	2%	40–65%	75%
Chance of kidney function deteriorating after the birth		20–50%	60%
Chance of severe kidney damage requiring dialysis or transplant		2–33%	40%

production in the ovaries) and periods. Generally speaking, the risks during pregnancy, for the health of the mother and baby, are less for women who have a well-functioning transplant. The table below shows the percentage chance of problems occurring for mothers who have a transplant, depending on the level of creatinine in the blood.

There is also a risk that the patient's transplant kidney may be damaged during the pregnancy; however, this too depends upon the patient's blood creatinine level when she gets pregnant. If the patient's blood creatinine is less than 100 µmol/l, the risk of damaging the transplant kidney is almost nil. However, if the patient's blood creatinine is between 100 and 130 µmol/l during the pregnancy, there is a 15% chance that the transplant will have failed after eight years. For women whose creatinine is more than 130 µmol/l when they become pregnant, there is a 35% chance that the transplant kidney will have failed after three years.

Kidney transplant patients who do get pregnant will be under the care of both the kidney and maternity teams. They will work together with the patient's GP and midwife throughout the pregnancy. It is important to monitor the kidney function and blood pressure during pregnancy. The drugs that transplant patients take to prevent rejection are unlikely to cause any problems during the pregnancy. Even so, it is best to tell your kidney doctor if you are planning to become pregnant, or as soon as you find out.

Once the baby is born, some of the drugs can be passed through breast milk, but many doctors feel that the benefits of breastfeeding the baby outweigh the risks.

Overall, if a woman with kidney failure wants to get pregnant, it is best for her to do so either in the early stages of kidney failure or after she has had a transplant (as long as it is working well). It should be pointed out that the baby is as likely as any other baby to be normal, and will not usually inherit the mother's condition. Nonetheless, any woman with kidney failure who is thinking about having a family should consider all the potential problems and risks, both for herself and for the baby, before going ahead. If she is in any doubt at all about whether to try for a baby, she should speak to the doctors and nurses in the kidney unit. They are there to

RISK OF PROBLEMS DURING PREGNANCY FOR KIDNEY TRANSPLANT PATIENTS

	Creatinine less than 120 µmol/l (CKF Stage 1)	Creatinine of more than 120 µmol/l (CKF Stages 2–5)
Chance of problems during pregnancy	30%	82%
Chance of a successful pregnancy	97%	75%
Chance of the mother having long-term health problems	7%	27%

help people make decisions like this.

If the risks are considered too great, some form of contraception is recommended. The Pill is best avoided in women who have high blood pressure or clotting problems. Other methods of contraception, such as the coil (intra-uterine device) or condoms, can be discussed with the doctor.

It is also a good idea to practise 'safe sex' by using condoms. This will reduce your risk of getting AIDS and other sexually transmitted diseases.

KEY FACTS

1 Sexual difficulties affect the majority of male and female dialysis patients.

2 You may find that doctors and nurses are reluctant to talk about sexual problems, and that it is down to you to raise the subject.

3 Erectile dysfunction (difficulty in getting or keeping a hard penis) is the most common and worrying problem for men with kidney failure.

4 Treatment of erectile dysfunction is usually successful, although you may need to be very patient.

5 Treating anaemia, adjusting the amount of dialysis and changing tablets can all help.

6 Viagra tablets have been shown to be effective in many dialysis patients, as have vacuum devices. Other tablets now available include Levitra and Cialis.

7 Other effective treatments include vacuum devices and penile insertion (transurethral) therapy.

8 Penile injection therapy may be successful, although there are disadvantages.

9 Sex and relationship counselling can be helpful. Talk to your doctor about whether you can be referred for this if you feel you and your partner would benefit.

10 Kidney failure affects women's periods. Pregnancy is less likely, but contraception is still needed.

11 A successful pregnancy is sometimes possible, but there are considerable risks for both mother and baby. It is important to discuss the risks with your doctor, if at all possible, before getting pregnant.

12 If you are a woman with kidney failure, and you want to have a baby, it is best for you to try to get pregnant either in the early stages of kidney failure or after a transplant, as long as the transplant is working well.

17 END OF LIFE CARE

This chapter explores some of those difficult issues around the subject of death and dying. The intention is to give readers the information necessary to make choices at the appropriate time – the best choices for them and those they love.

INTRODUCTION

Death is a subject seldom discussed openly with patients in a dialysis unit. Dialysis and kidney transplants represent, after all, the success of our knowledge and skill in conquering a previously fatal illness. These treatments are *all about life*. Yet nobody can attend a kidney unit without the realisation that death is always close at hand. In a large dialysis centre, a week rarely passes without someone dying. Units are close communities, where patients know many of those attending as friends. Each of them will be aware, therefore, of a succession of losses, reminding them of the fragility of their own lives.

People with kidney failure live with the knowledge that they have a shorter life expectancy than the rest of the population (as can be seen from the tables in *Chapter 18*). The cause of death is not usually kidney failure, with the exception of one important group – those who choose not to receive dialysis. We feel it is right, therefore, to include a chapter in this book, acknowledging the fact that what doctors can provide is far from perfect.

There is no doubt that life on dialysis can be full, rewarding and worthwhile for many people. However, there are some who feel either that they would not wish to live with the limitations imposed by treatment, or that they have done so long enough. When the need for dialysis approaches, those who are already elderly, or whose lives are seriously restricted by other illnesses, may decide that they would rather allow nature to 'take its course' – even though this means they will die. Some, therefore, choose not to start dialysis treatment. There are others, who may have dialysed for many years, becoming more frail or disabled as time goes on, who decide that the time has come to stop treatment and die with dignity.

It is important for patients and their families to understand that dialysis is not compulsory. If you do not wish to receive treatment, or decide that you wish to stop dialysis, you should discuss this with the staff at your renal unit. Not having dialysis treatment will mean that the patient will die, usually within a few days or weeks, depending on their degree of kidney failure. Patients and their families are the only people that can judge whether quality of life with dialysis is acceptable. You may be frail or elderly, severely disabled or restricted, yet satisfied that life is still worthwhile.

Most units have a sympathetic attitude and will offer you all the information and support you need in taking this decision.

DEATH FROM KIDNEY FAILURE

Patients are often afraid to ask renal unit staff, whose lives are devoted to maintaining life against the odds, what it is like to die from kidney failure. While every death is different (just as every life is different), it can be said with some confidence that it is, in general, 'not a bad way to go'. The problems that occur in the final days of death from kidney failure vary from person to person. The symptoms that may need to be controlled include feeling sick (nausea), muscle twitching and breathlessness. Sometimes there is some agitation and confusion. Pain is not usually a serious problem.

Nausea can be caused by the waste products, usually removed by normal kidneys, building up in the blood. There are several drugs available that can be used to reduce or prevent nausea. Breathlessness may be due to fluid overload. Both drugs and suction treatment can be used to keep the lungs clear to reduce breathlessness, while carefully administered drug treatment can keep the patient comfortable and free from distress. Most of the drugs used for nausea, breathlessness or agitation (e.g. morphine and similar drugs) cause some degree of sedation, leading to drowsiness.

Patients and families usually want to know how long a person can survive with untreated ERF. This too is variable, depending on the extent to which their old kidneys are working – and therefore the amount of urine that they pass. The kidneys may be able to get rid of some excess fluid, but unable to process waste products such as creatinine and urea, or salts such as potassium. It is the build-up of these substances in the blood (especially the potassium) that usually leads to death.

On average, patients who are passing reasonable amounts of urine (say over 1 litre per day) can survive for about 2–6 weeks. If little or no urine is passed, they may survive for 10–14 days. During this period, they generally become increasingly weak and drowsy, sleep more and more, and finally become unconscious. Then they will pass away peacefully.

WHERE SHOULD THIS PERIOD BE SPENT?

This is very much up to the individual and family. If a patient wishes to be at home, specialist nursing can be arranged through the GP. It is very important for some people to feel they are in familiar surroundings, with family members and pets around them. Whenever this is the case, people with ERF should receive every support to spend their last days at home.

Some hospices (which mainly deal with patients dying from cancer) will admit kidney patients who have decided to stop dialysis or not to start it in the first place. Hospice care and support of the dying is particularly sympathetic, taking into account the needs and feelings of both patient and family.

Most kidney units are experienced in the care of dying patients, who are usually nursed in a side ward, offering quiet and privacy. It is usual for relatives to be allowed to stay with the patient all the time. Some kidney units offer accommodation in a 'relatives' room'. One of the benefits of remaining in hospital is that, if the person has a change of heart and decides to go for dialysis after all, the facilities are close at hand.

THE DECISION NOT TO START DIALYSIS TREATMENT

If a person attending a pre-dialysis clinic tells the kidney consultant that, when the need arises, he or she does not want dialysis treatment, it is important that this decision is made with full knowledge – it is an 'informed' choice.

In the first place, the patient needs to ask the doctor, quite directly, about the likely outcome – i.e. how long they might expect to live both with and without dialysis, and also what can be done to make their last days comfortable if they choose not to dialyse. This information is essential for making a rational decision. It may be that, with dietary care and medication, a person would live for some months, free of frequent hospital visits or preparations for treatment such as access surgery. This is particularly true in the case of very elderly people, leading an inactive life.

We do not know that dialysis necessarily prolongs the life of all very frail elderly people (especially those over, say, 80 years of age). This does not mean they will not be offered the treatment. If dialysis does prolong life a little, then the quality of that life could be poorer than it would have been had dialysis not been started. One research study looking at frail elderly patients found that the average length of survival on dialysis was 8 months, whereas a similar population without dialysis could expect to live for 6 months. In other words, dialysis prolonged the patients' lives by 2 months. In addition to this, most of the patients who did receive dialysis spent a high proportion of their 8 months in hospital, and many died in hospital. The majority of the other (non-dialysis group) on the other hand, died at home.

It is important to be aware too that it is impossible to know exactly what life on dialysis is like unless one has experienced it. Even talking to others receiving treatment does not give the full picture, as everyone is different. Sometimes, patients agree to treatment reluctantly, only to find that it is not nearly as bad as they had imagined it would be. Others tell us that, on the contrary, they had expected it to be much easier to cope with, or that they had hoped to feel far better on treatment than they actually do.

Having dialysis will prolong life in most (but not all) people, so weighing up the risks and benefits of not having treatment is very important for each individual.

TRIALS OF DIALYSIS

To discover what life on dialysis is like, some patients opt for a 'trial of dialysis', lasting a few weeks or months. This allows them to discover both the good and bad sides of life on dialysis, and to decide whether the benefits outweigh the drawbacks.

In some cases, a short period of treatment may be undertaken in order to give patients time to settle their affairs, or resolve conflicting feelings in the family. These are not uncommon during the heightened emotional tension surrounding such a decision. Others need time to allow visits from family members living abroad, and to say goodbye. Everything should be done that will allow the patient peace of mind. Relatives, too, need a sense of resolution, free from unnecessary guilt and regret.

CHOOSING THE LESSER OF TWO EVILS

There may be good medical reasons to decide not to dialyse, without even considering a trial of treatment. If a patient with kidney failure is already suffering from another terminal illness, for example an inoperable cancer, a progressive brain or blood vessel disease (such as recurrent strokes) or severe heart failure, it can be a blessing in disguise to be offered the opportunity of refusing dialysis. This can allow a dignified death, in less distressing circumstances than might otherwise apply. Those who need dialysis to stay alive have a control over the time and manner of their death that is denied to most other people.

THOSE WHO CANNOT MAKE AN INFORMED CHOICE

So far, we have only considered those people who are in a position to make an informed choice. Sadly, some patients may have a condition or illness that makes it impossible for them to choose what they wish to do. Those with advanced dementia (with Alzheimer's disease, for example) or severe learning difficulties may not be able to understand the implications of the decision. They might, in addition, be unable to understand the necessity of attending for dialysis, or of observing diet and fluid restriction – and would, in all probability, find the treatment very hard to tolerate. Each case needs to be considered on its merits, with the patient's best interests always in mind.

People who have had a stroke causing irreversible brain damage, or an illness or injury that makes them drowsy or semi-conscious all the time, cannot express an opinion about their wishes. In these cases, it is much more difficult for the doctors to know how to act for the best – i.e. in the patient's best interests. It can be helpful, especially for the relatives, if people with kidney failure make their wishes known at a time when they are able to decide for themselves.

If you feel that there are circumstances in which you would not wish to be kept alive by dialysis, you can confirm this in writing, and ask for the document to be kept in your medical notes. While this document, sometimes called a 'Living Will' or an 'Advanced Directive', has no legal status, it is valuable in giving a guide to your doctor and next of kin, and in reducing any feelings of guilt your family may experience after your death.

Most kidney consultants will discuss all the options with the family, the patient's GP, the multidisciplinary team in the unit, and any others close to the patient. The consultant has the final responsibility for deciding what is in the best interests of the patient, having taken everyone's views into consideration.

THE DECISION TO STOP DIALYSIS

Withdrawal from dialysis is not an uncommon cause of death in long-standing dialysis patients, particularly those who are elderly. In fact, up to 20% of patients die in this way.

For some people, dialysis can become like a treadmill, or a conveyor belt, on which they feel as if they are trapped. The truth is that nobody can force a patient to attend for dialysis. To dialyse somebody against his or her will is legally an 'assault'.

Sometimes, the very knowledge that they are able to stop when they wish is enough to give individuals the will to carry on for the present.

Patients sometimes fear that they are 'letting down' the staff of the kidney unit by wanting to stop treatment. It can seem like ingratitude, or a rejection of the care they have been given. While staff will be sad, they may also be relieved, having been aware of the person's distress. They should, in any case, respect the patient's decision. Nobody can know fully what life is like for another person.

There are many reasons why this decision may be taken. Probably the most common is that the patient suffers a medical setback, often unrelated to the kidneys, such as a stroke. In patients with diabetes, needing to have a limb amputated would be such a setback. It would inevitably result in further disability and limitation, which the patient might regard as just too much to cope with. Life on dialysis may have been tolerable, but the additional problem may remove what quality remained in the patient's life. Loss of independence is often the deciding factor.

The second most common reason for withdrawal is the gradual deterioration caused by ageing and the complications of many years of dialysis. The patient may have considerable pain and restriction from renal bone disease, or problems with blood circulation from narrowing of the arteries.

Dialysis access may have become difficult over the years, leading to frequent hospital admissions. Older patients may also have been bereaved due to the death of their spouse, resulting in less motivation to carry on for the sake of others. Whatever the reasons, the person may feel that it is no longer worth the struggle to continue.

If a patient asks renal unit staff to discontinue dialysis, the subject should be gently explored, to see whether there is anything that can be done to improve the situation. In some people, the request to withdraw is a cry for help, or an expression of a state of depression that could be helped either by sympathetic counselling or by medication. In some cases, patients may be asked to talk things over with a counsellor, psychologist or psychiatrist, to discover whether this is the case. Stopping dialysis is a decision that should not be rushed, but properly considered. Some patients wish to stop, but find their families become distressed by the suggestion. It is important that the feelings of the others who are involved are considered and explored, but the final decision should be the patient's alone.

WITHDRAWING FROM TREATMENT AFTER TRANSPLANT

While successful transplantation offers the best possible quality of life for a patient with kidney failure, it is not without risks. The powerful drugs used to prevent rejection can lead to infections, skin cancers and, in a minority of cases, more serious cancers, especially lymphoma. There is growing concern that newer, stronger drugs which are better at preventing rejection may also be 'better' at stopping the immune system from preventing cancer. It is possible, therefore, that cancer is becoming more common in patients on these drugs. Patients need to be aware of the risks as well as the benefits of transplantation and to discuss their concerns with their consultant. (More information about the risks of transplantation can be found in *Chapter 13*.)

One of the treatments for some serious types of cancer (including lymphoma) is to stop (or reduce the doses of) the immuno-suppressant drugs. In this case, the kidney may be rejected and the patient will need to go back onto dialysis. If the cancer is so advanced that no measures will prevent it, the patient is left with a bleak decision. Life might be prolonged for a short time by stopping the immuno-suppressant drugs and returning to dialysis. But this involves more time spent in hospital when time is short in any case. The advantage of being on dialysis is that the patient can choose when

they've had enough, and decide to withdraw. Some patients, however, feel it is preferable to continue the immuno-suppressant drugs and maintain the kidney, but allow the cancer to take a quicker course. Should you be unlucky enough to find yourself in this situation, your doctors should be able to guide you as to the best decision in your particular case.

Other patients, who have had a long period of successful transplantation, develop an incurable condition not related to the drugs they are taking. These patients have a range of options which their doctor should discuss with them. One option might be to stop taking their immuno-suppressant medicine and allow the kidney to reject (and fail). Then they could die from kidney failure without dialysis, if the death from kidney failure is 'better' than it would have been from their new incurable disease. Or, if the incurable disease is killing them slowly, they might decide not to have dialysis when their transplant 'naturally' fails at a later date.

There is another group of patients, often elderly ones, who are not dying of an incurable disease. But the build-up of serious although non-fatal complications of kidney failure (such as bone pain or 'access' problems) is becoming too much for them. So they can 'take the opportunity' of their transplant's 'natural failure' to allow themselves to die, rather than suffer a new period of dialysis – especially when they know they are now unfit to have another transplant and would otherwise have to have dialysis until they die anyway.

SPIRITUAL CONCERNS

Those who do not wish to receive dialysis or stop treatment after receiving it sometimes express concerns that this is the equivalent of suicide, and therefore against the teachings of most major religions. The same views might also be expressed by patients who allow their transplants to fail then refuse dialysis. However, leaders from a number of different faiths have considered the case of the kidney patient who wishes to withdraw from treatment, and none has concluded that such withdrawal is either suicidal or sinful. The basis for this is that, but for an artificial and highly technological treatment, the patient would have died naturally in the first place. One could see this as the original decree of fate, nature or the Deity. As a result of human intervention, the patient has lived beyond his or her natural term. To give up dialysis or stop taking immuno-suppressant drugs is simply to cease prolonging life unnaturally in someone whose body is not capable of sustaining itself.

Any patient, or relative of a patient, who has any concerns, or needs spiritual support, should talk to his or her priest or religious leader. Many hospitals now have a chaplaincy service, with leaders from all the major faiths available to give support and advice.

KEY FACTS

1 Dialysis is not compulsory. A trial of treatment may be a sensible option, while you are making up your mind.

2 Withdrawal from dialysis is not uncommon, especially in older patients.

3 The reason for withdrawal is usually a medical event unrelated to the kidneys – such as a stroke or cancer.

4 The decision should not be rushed, allowing time for others to come to terms with the situation.

5 Death from renal failure need not be distressing, if well managed. It should take place where the patient feels most comfortable.

6 The wish to stop dialysis may be due to depression, or a cry for help, needing action to improve some intolerable situation.

7 Kidney patients have greater control in ensuring a dignified death than most other people.

8 Where a patient is not capable of an informed choice, the consultant has the final responsibility, after discussion with everybody concerned.

9 Transplant patients can decide to stop their immuno-suppressant drugs, to make them reject and lose the kidney, and then not have dialysis. In this way, they can allow themselves to die of kidney failure.

10 Refusing dialysis, or deliberately allowing a transplant to fail, is not suicide. A patient who wishes to take this route should not be made to feel guilty.

11 If religion is important to a patient, it is a good idea for them to discuss these issues with a priest or other religious leader – either from their own community or from the hospital.

18 STATISTICS AND OUTCOMES

This chapter looks at the effect of kidney failure on a patient's life expectancy. It goes on to consider the levels of care available to kidney patients in the UK and in other countries, and how this is likely to change in the future.

INTRODUCTION

The number of patients being treated for kidney failure in the UK has increased in recent years. Without dialysis or a transplant anyone with established renal failure (ERF) will die within a few weeks. With successful treatment, some people with ERF can expect to live for many years. However, it is still true that not enough patients in the UK are getting the treatment they need. This is the case for both dialysis and transplantation, and the latter part of the chapter considers some of the reasons why this might be.

SURVIVAL WITH KIDNEY FAILURE

Kidney function is essential for life. Once a person's own kidneys fail, some form of treatment is necessary if they are to go on living. Currently there are two forms of treatment – dialysis (in which the kidney function is taken over by artificial means), and transplant (in which another person's kidney is used instead). Successful treatment – by dialysis or a transplant – now gives people with kidney failure a new lease of life, sometimes for many years. But how many years?

PERCENTAGE SURVIVAL FOR PEOPLE ON DIALYSIS, ACCORDING TO AGE AT START OF DIALYSIS

Years	1	2	3	4	5	10
Age 18-64:	88.5	81.4	75.5	70.0	64.9	42.6
Age 65+:	65.9	51.4	40.9	32.7	25.3	3.9
All ages	76.9	65.9	57.6	50.6	44.2	26.0

Source: Renal Registry, 2007

The 'Survival on Dialysis according to age' table above shows the percentage chances of still being alive one, two, three, four, five and ten years after the start of dialysis. People who start dialysis when they are young clearly have a better chance of surviving for longer than people who start dialysis later in life. Perhaps this point is not surprising, given that older people are more likely to die than younger people when they do not have kidney failure. However, people on dialysis have much less chance of surviving for 5 years than healthy people in the same age group.

This data is worrying, especially when you look at patients in early to middle-life. As you can see, people in the 'younger age group' (18 – 64 yrs) have only a 65% chance of being alive after five years of the diagnosis of ERF. This outlook is worse than for most types of cancer.

LIFE EXPECTANCY (IN YEARS) AT DIFFERENT AGE GROUPS

Age	Life expectancy (yrs)	ERF
0–14	71	20
15–19	62	18
20–24	57	15
25–29	52	13
30–34	47	11
35–39	43	10
40–44	38	9
45–49	34	7
50–54	29	7
54–59	25	6
60–64	21	5
65–69	17	4
70–74	14	3
75–79	11	3
80–84	8	2
85+	4	2

(Source: USRDS 2009)

Conversely, you could argue that the data for the later years (65+) is not too bad, with 66% surviving one year, and 25% five years. People in this age group may well consider this gain in life worth having.

Another way of looking at survival is to look at the average number of years a person is likely to live, after the start of dialysis, and comparing it to the life expectancy of the population as a whole. This is summarised in the table on the left.

In other words, ERF has a major impact on life expectancy, especially in younger people (20–44 years), reducing it fourfold. In fact, if you look through all the age groups, there is about a fourfold difference in life expectancy. But an older patient (for example, from the 75–79 age group) may be very grateful for the three years (on average) of life they may gain, so there is every reason to offer dialysis to the older person.

These figures include all patients, whatever the cause of their kidney failure, but the life expectancy will be higher in patients with a 'good-outlook' cause of ERF, (glomerulonephritis and polycystic kidney disease), and lower in a 'bad-outlook' cause (e.g. diabetes, myeloma, amyloidosis and renovascular disease).

WHY DO PEOPLE WITH KIDNEY FAILURE DIE?

Although people with kidney failure have a lower than average life expectancy, once they start treatment (by either dialysis or a transplant) they are more likely to die from something other than kidney disease. The most common reason that people with kidney failure die is because they have heart disease as well. As can be seen from the table *on page 135*, 29% of patients with kidney failure die of heart problems.

Perhaps this is not surprising as, in most developed countries, a large number of people in the population as a whole (about 30%) die of heart disease. Interestingly, there are fewer deaths from stroke and cancer than you might expect. The fewer deaths than expected from cancer is surprising as cancer is overall more common in both dialysis and transplant patients – in fact three times more common than expected in transplant patients. This is because, even though cancer is more common, it is not what dialysis and transplant patients die from. In other words, often they die (for example, of a heart problem) with cancer rather than from it.

There are also other causes of death among kidney patients. For example, 15% of UK patients with advanced kidney failure die because they choose to stop dialysis. This and the surrounding issues are discussed fully in Chapter 17. Also many people with kidney failure die of infections (18% of patients in the UK). Dialysis patients may be prone to peritonitis or infections of access sites (*see page 65; 75–6*). In transplant patients, infections occur because the patient is taking immuno-suppressant drugs (*see page 99*) to prevent rejection of the kidney.

Meanwhile, common sense tells us that the general state of a patient's health will also have a bearing on how long that person will live. Everyone, whether or not they have kidney failure, will be at greater risk of dying early if they have had a heart attack or stroke, peripheral vascular disease (narrowing of the arteries to the legs), serious cancers and diabetes. If someone with kidney failure has none of these conditions, they have a good chance of long-term survival, either on dialysis or with a transplant.

People are more likely to die from the complications of kidney failure, especially those affecting the heart, than from the kidney failure itself. It seems that permanent damage to the heart often occurs early in kidney failure, before dialysis or a transplant is needed. This damage is probably due to several factors, including high blood pressure, anaemia and fluid overload. It is also possible that the wastes that build up in the blood in people with kidney failure have a directly toxic effect on the heart. Neither dialysis nor a transplant can do anything to repair an already damaged heart.

INDIVIDUALS NOT STATISTICS

Although statistics can give an indication of the average survival chances of different groups of patients treated for kidney failure, they cannot predict what will happen to any one person. People with kidney failure are individuals not statistics. Even if you belong to a group of patients whose overall chance of survival is poor, you as an individual may still survive for many years. Your survival odds are obviously better if you belong to one of the groups with the best chances of survival.

HOW GOOD ARE THE SERVICES AROUND THE WORLD?

Survival is affected by two things – the severity of a person's disease and the treatment services that are available. While dialysis and transplantation can make an enormous difference to a person's life expectancy, the availability of these treatments does vary from one country to another. One way of assessing how good the services for kidney patients are, is to make comparisons with the services available in other countries.

In order to make useful comparisons about what treatment is available to kidney patients in different

THE MOST COMMON CAUSES OF DEATH IN PEOPLE WITH KIDNEY FAILURE

Heart disease	29%
Infection	18%
Treatment stopped	15%
Cancer	8%
Strokes	5%
Others	10%
Uncertain	16%

Source: Renal Registry (2007)

A COMPARISON OF THE NUMBER OF PEOPLE NEWLY DIAGNOSED WITH KIDNEY FAILURE AND RECEIVING TREATMENT IN SEVERAL COUNTRIES (PMP)

Country		2000	2001	2002	2003	2004	2005	2006	2007
1	Taiwan	323	357	365	391	405	435	420	415
2	Mexico				280	346	302	346	372
3	USA	325	328	336	343	347	354	365	361
4	Japan	252	252	262	263	267	271	275	285
5	Turkey	115	141	122	112	121	179	192	229
6	Luxembourg				180	188	166	224	
7	Germany	175	184	174	186	194	203	213	
8	Israel				188	189	186	192	193
9	Greece	157	164	165	180	197	194	197	190
10	Belgium (Dutch)			170	175	181	183	193	186
11	Czech Rep				167	166	175	186	185
12	Korea (Rep)				152	171	173	185	184
13	Canada	143	152	154	162	163	163	163	
14	Thailand				78	123	110	139	159
15	Argentina					137	140	141	151
16	Austria	133	136	132	140	161	154	159	151
17	Hungary	129	130		139	139	162	159	151
18	Bosnia Herz		77	95	166	108	104	133	151
19	Hong Kong				128	141	145	149	147
20	Chile				130	157	135	141	144
21	Croatia				131	155	144		
22	Malaysia				106	114	121	137	143

countries, it is necessary to take population size into account. This is done by dividing yearly totals from a particular country by the number of millions of people in that country's population. This provides us with tables of comparable figures expressed as numbers per million population (pmp).

The table above shows the numbers of people diagnosed with kidney failure and starting treatment (by either dialysis or transplant) over several years in different countries. As can be seen, the UK has one of the lowest rates of starting patients on dialysis in the developed world.

In healthcare, as in football, some countries are clearly better than others. If all football teams were equally good, all teams would gain the same number of points each year – and all would come 'equal top'. Every world cup match would end in a draw. However, not everyone can be top all or even some of the time, and there may be a number of reasons why any country holds the position it does.

A COMPARISON OF THE NUMBER OF PEOPLE NEWLY DIAGNOSED WITH KIDNEY FAILURE AND RECEIVING TREATMENT IN SEVERAL COUNTRIES (PMP) *continued*

Country	2000	2001	2002	2003	2004	2005	2006	2007
23 Uruguay	121	124		146	151	146	138	143
24 Denmark			130	132	131	121	119	140
25 France						139	140	138
26 Sweden	126	124	125	122	123	121	130	129
27 Poland	68	84	99	103	97	120	122	127
28 Spain	132	127	126		175	126	128	121
29 Italy	131	136	142	133	161	121		
30 Netherlands	93	101	100	103	106	107	112	118
31 Norway	89	95	92	96	101	99	100	113
32 Australia	92	97	94	100	97	113	118	110
33 New Zealand	110	119	115	115	113	112	118	109
34 UK		**89**	**95**	**101**	**91**	**101**	**105**	**106**
35 Finland	90	91	94	95	97	97	87	92
36 Philippines				60	75	79	80	92
37 Romania						94	75	90
38 Iceland				73	79	67	69	81
39 Iran				61	71	72	66	
40 Pakistan				32		22	29	
41 Russia				19	17	24	28	
42 Bangladesh				8	7	8	8	13

Source: Adapted from USRDS 2009

The table shows that Taiwan and the United States have three times as many people per million population with ERF, than the UK. One possible explanation is that people from different countries are not similar – that people who live in the UK are not genetically predisposed to developing kidney failure, while Taiwanese and North Americans are. This is unlikely.

A possible reason for the variation in numbers of people being treated is that some countries are better than others at identifying and providing treatment for people who develop kidney failure.

The fact that countries such as Taiwan and the USA have much higher numbers of patients on dialysis than the UK suggests that the UK is failing to treat large numbers of people who develop kidney failure. This is all the more worrying when it is remembered that many people with ERF die within a few weeks unless they are treated by dialysis or a transplant.

Fortunately for kidney patients in the UK, the rate at which patients are starting dialysis is improving (as you can see if you read across the UK row, on the table), but the rate of improvement is still too slow.

INTERNATIONAL RATES OF TRANSPLANTATION

It is not just in dialysis that there are major differences in service around the world. The opportunity to have a transplant is also very variable.

A way of assessing how well different countries are meeting the need for treatment for kidney failure is to compare the number of kidney patients with a functioning transplant. Like the rate for dialysis (see page 136), the rate of kidney transplantation should be similar in all countries. Again, this is far from being the case. Some countries perform many more kidney transplants than others.

The UK's rate of 25 transplants per million population (pmp) places it 28th of 42 countries where we know the transplant rate. Norway and Spain are the 'transplant kings' each with twice the transplant rate of the UK. Norway and Spain achieve good results in two different ways. Norway makes sure that all potential living donors are informed about the possibility of helping their loved one. And indeed, they find that if they do this, many more do come forward to donate. Spain, on the other hand, emphasises deceased donor transplantation. One way they do this is to have transplant co-ordinators in every main hospital in the land, so that all potential donors are assessed.

UK POSTCODE LOTTERY IN TRANSPLANTATION

As well as being well down the 'World Transplant League', we have major problems within our country too. In the UK, it is by no means true that all transplant centres have the same results – as can be seen from the table on the right. In terms of the likelihood of the kidney working five years after the transplant, there is a 16% difference from the top to the bottom of the table.

There are huge differences in terms of the likelihood of one unit carrying out a living donor transplant. In one unit in London, 7% of transplanted kidneys are from

Hospital	5 yr kidney Deceased donor	% Living transplants	Waiting time for Deceased donor transplants survival (days)
Coventry	90	67	1628
St George's, London	88	16	915
Oxford	87	22	872
Bristol	87	36	1010
West London	87	28	1524
Cardiff	85	28	860
Cambridge	83	22	864
Portsmouth	83	31	876
London/Barts	83	8	1255
Edinburgh	83	25	1443
Sheffield	83	30	1547
UK	**82**	**36**	**1110**
Newcastle	82	33	570
Guy's, London	82	32	1062
Royal Free, London	81	7	1001
Manchester	81	28	1169
Birmingham	81	41	1484
Liverpool	80	25	926
Glasgow	80	34	1329
Nottingham	80	34	1600
Leeds	79	28	782
Belfast	79	21	1737
Leicester	75	60	1825
Plymouth	74	29	716

Source: UK Transplant, 2008 (2006-2008 data)

living donors, way below the national average of 36%. What is probably most worrying is the country's very long average wait for a deceased donor kidney. It is 1110 days – just over three years; with a huge range from 570 days in Newcastle to 1825 days in Leicester.

In the next chapter, we look at what policies are being put in place to make sure that good care is shared out fairly around the country. We also look at ways in which people with kidney failure can take control of their own care, and their own lives.

KEY FACTS

1 Without dialysis or a transplant, people die within a few weeks of developing ERF. Successful treatment (by dialysis or a transplant) can prolong life for many years.

2 Even with treatment survival is poor, with about 77% surviving one year, 44% surviving 5 years, and 26% surviving 10 years.

3 ERF has a significant effect on life expectancy. Someone aged between 35 and 39 can expect to live a further 10 years compared to 43 years of additional life expectancy for the general, healthy population.

4 Average survival chances for people on dialysis (or after a transplant) are affected by age, the underlying cause of kidney failure and various other medical factors.

5 People with kidney failure are individuals not statistics. Doctors cannot predict for sure what will happen to any one person and that includes you.

6 Some countries treat a far higher proportion of their people who develop kidney failure than do others.

7 The number of people per million population in the UK who are having treatment for kidney failure is much lower than it should be.

8 There is a serious shortfall in the provision of treatment – both dialysis and transplantation – for kidney failure throughout the UK.

9 The UK still suffers from a transplantation 'postcode lottery' – i.e. where you live in the UK can affect how long you are likely to wait for a transplant, how easy it will be for you to have a living donor transplant, and how long your new kidney will last.

19 NEW DEVELOPMENTS AND CHOICE

The final chapter of this book looks at the developments in the delivery of care to patients with kidney failure throughout the UK. It considers the factors that affect patients' choice.

INTRODUCTION

The figures given in the previous chapter show UK services for kidney patients as ranking well behind those of many other countries in the developed world. There are a number of reasons why this could be the case. Two factors are particularly important: there are too few renal units and too few kidney transplants being carried out.

THE NUMBER OF RENAL UNITS

One reason why the provision of treatment for kidney failure in the UK is so low is because this country has relatively few renal units (and therefore relatively few specialist kidney doctors, nurses and other specialist healthcare workers). This has an impact on the number of patients that can be treated and the number of new patients that are referred for treatment.

In 2000, as part of the NHS Plan, the government announced substantial funding for Renal Services in the UK. They promised that by 2004 there would be 450 new haemodialysis stations available to treat up to 1850 extra patients. To finance this expansion, they invested £18 million in renal services during 2001–2003. Despite this extra money, Renal Services still don't appear to be able to keep up with demand. The main problem is that kidney failure is relatively expensive to treat. Although it only affects about 0.05% of the UK population, 1.5% of the healthcare budget is spent on treating kidney failure. It is obvious therefore that other ways need to be found to increase the number of patients that can be treated in the UK. Relatively little use is made of home-based dialysis therapies, such as PD, which can be more cost effective than hospital or satellite-based haemodialysis. Transplantation is the most cost effective treatment and is also under utilised, for a number of reasons.

THE NUMBER OF KIDNEY TRANSPLANTS

In the UK there are not enough transplant operations performed to keep up with demand. There are a number of possible sources of kidneys for transplantation – deceased donor, living donor and non-heart beating donor. The most common source of kidneys is from deceased donors. However, over recent years, improvements in road safety, seat belt laws and better healthcare have meant that the number of kidneys that become available for transplantation has decreased. The

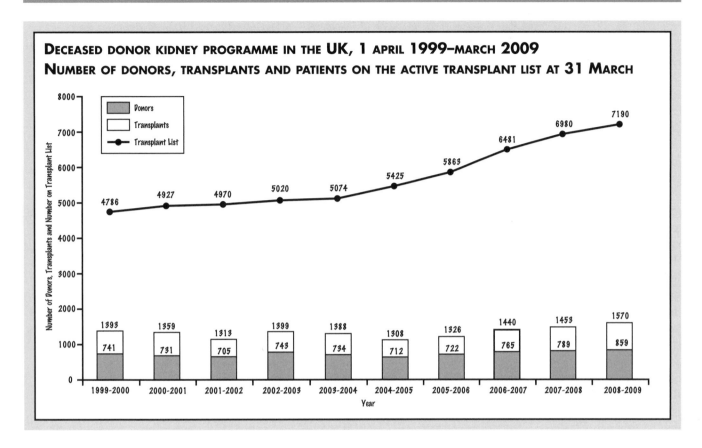

DECEASED DONOR KIDNEY PROGRAMME IN THE UK, 1 APRIL 1999–MARCH 2009

NUMBER OF DONORS, TRANSPLANTS AND PATIENTS ON THE ACTIVE TRANSPLANT LIST AT 31 MARCH

situation would be improved if more people registered their willingness to donate their organs for transplantation and discussed their wishes with their next of kin.

Even more important is the lack of beds in Intensive Care Units (ICUs) in the UK. If a patient becomes brain dead, and therefore a potential ('heart-beating') kidney donor, that person needs to be kept on a life-support machine to preserve their organs (including their kidneys) until an operation can be performed to remove them. When ICU beds are in short supply, patients who have a chance of recovery must be given priority over patients who are already brain dead. Inevitably, many potential deceased donor organs are lost in this way. Also,

relatively few units have a 'non-heart beating' donor programme (*see Chapter 12* on Living donor transplants).

As not enough deceased donor transplants are being done, it would make most sense to increase the number of living related (and unrelated) donor transplants, especially as this is the best and most cost effective treatment for ERF.

One possible reason why a patient may not be given a living related transplant is that they think they have no medically suitable donors among their family members. In fact, medical unsuitability among family members is relatively uncommon.

Carrying out a living related or unrelated transplant requires a lot of preparation work by renal doctors, nurses and transplant co-ordinators. Not all renal units in the UK put much time and effort into such work, finding it generally 'easier' (less work) to put patients on the 'normal' (deceased donor) transplant waiting list. Also carrying out transplants from living people means that doctors and nurses are more likely to have to confront 'difficult' issues with patients and their relatives. Perhaps some prefer to avoid this altogether.

The low rate of transplantation from living donors that we have seen across the UK so far, is partly the fault of the doctors and nurses who don't always tell patients and their relatives, partners and friends about the full range of possibilities. If potential donors are not told that kidney donation is a possibility, and are not gently encouraged to come forward, they are unlikely to do so. But donating a kidney to a friend or family member can be more complicated than you think, in all sorts of ways. This will be particularly true if your relationship is not an easy one to start with.

You can see from the table in Chapter 18 (*page 138*) that there are vast differences in the number of living transplants done throughout the UK. For example, if you are living in Coventry, Bristol, Birmingham or Leicester, you are more likely to be encouraged to have a living donor transplant than if, say, you were living in parts of London, Belfast or Liverpool.

It is interesting to note that the number of living donor transplants done in the UK does not seem to have an impact on the overall number of transplants that are performed. So even if the unit down the road from you is doing more living donor transplants, it doesn't mean that you are any more likely to get a transplant (from any source, living or deceased donor). In fact the number of people on the waiting list for a transplant continues to rise at a much faster rate than the rate of increase in the number of transplants performed. This can be seen by the graph on page 141 which shows the number of deceased donor transplants that are performed each year and the number of patients waiting for a transplant each year. More information about this subject can be found on the NHS Blood and Transplant website (*see page 163*).

CHOICE – REAL OR NOT?

During the early part of the twenty-first century a buzzword has crept into the minds of UK citizens . . . 'choice'. The government wants the people of this country to have a choice of public services: whether that is for transport, schools or hospitals (including Renal Units).

Through the use of the Internet, the press, data collected by organisations such as Ofsted (who report on schools' performance) and the 'Star system' in hospitals, it is now relatively easy to find out where better services are available. This system obviously attracts more pupils, customers or patients to the better performing services. The better units will hopefully drive up the standards of the less good, and the public will get the best for themselves and their family.

However, the matter of choice is far more complicated than it might first appear when it comes to the provision of services for the treatment of kidney failure. There are a huge number of factors that affect your choices, some of which are within your control and some, unfortunately which are not.

Availability of resources

As discussed above, there are clearly very different levels of service provided in various parts of the UK. In some areas, you are more likely to be encouraged to have a living donor transplant than in others. Additionally, there are very few renal units in the UK which encourage patients to have home haemodialysis. On average, about 47% of dialysis patients are treated with hospital-based haemodialysis, 31% in a satellite HD unit, 2% with home HD and 20% with home-based PD. However, in some hospitals as few as 6% of patients have a home-based treatment, either PD or HD. This begs the question whether all kidney patients in the UK actually get a choice of all forms of dialysis treatment or if treatments are offered depending on the services that are available. If hospital or satellite-based haemodialysis facilities exist in an area, it makes financial sense to have them operating at full capacity.

It is possible for patients to move house so that they live close to a renal unit that is able to offer them their treatment of choice, but this is impractical for most people.

Time

The amount of time a person has before they start treatment for kidney failure can have a big impact on their 'choice' of treatment. People who are referred to a renal unit months or years before treatment is needed, are far more likely to be given a full programme of education in small frequent sessions. They will be able to go away and think about the information they have been given, ask questions and make informed choices. People who arrive on a renal unit requiring dialysis immediately, however, are much more likely to be offered no choice of treatment and to be started on haemodialysis, usually with temporary access (*see page 70*) which carries a high risk of infection.

It is also true that patients who are referred to the renal unit in plenty of time are much more likely to have a kidney transplant before they actually need dialysis, particularly if they are being treated at a hospital where they actively encourage living donor transplants. However, there are some hospitals that never offer a transplant to a patient before they have started dialysis.

Social circumstances

A person's social situation may also affect their choice of treatment. For example, home dialysis (either PD or haemodialysis) requires some storage space and most people who have home haemodialysis also need some support from a helper.

People who work or do a lot of travelling may choose PD in preference to haemodialysis. However, if you live very close to a renal unit, hospital or satellite-based haemodialysis might be the treatment of choice for you, purely for reasons of convenience.

Education, information and decision making

If patients are to be offered a true choice of treatment, then that choice should be an informed one. Therefore education and information are vital to the decision making process. In order for patients to receive useful information it should be done in a way that is appropriate for each individual. Some people learn well through reading books and leaflets, others like to use the Internet and some like to watch videos. Many prefer to talk to a healthcare professional or another patient to gain their experience. It's therefore important for the people who are giving the information to be aware of how you like to learn.

People who are diagnosed with kidney failure in good time may spend many years visiting the renal clinic. Each time they visit, they may see a different doctor. Each doctor could have different levels of experience, which could make their opinions biased against one treatment or another. For example, doctors who have little or no experience of PD (usually because they work within the hospital and PD patients are generally at home, particularly if they are well) may give quite a negative impression of PD.

Once a patient has been given all of the relevant education, it is important for them to review the information is a systematic way so that an informed decision can be made. This can be done by listing the pros and cons for each treatment on a sheet of paper, or by looking at how each treatment option will impact on their life. The decision about the right treatment is unique for each patient, as everyone has different needs and expectations at different times in their life. No two patients are the same, and even for the same patient, there may be a reason why one treatment might be more suitable than another at different times in their life.

Making the right decision can be difficult, but it is important to remember that throughout your life with kidney failure, you may experience all types of treatment. The more information you have, the easier it will be to make the right choice at the right time. We hope that this book has given you some information that will help, and the confidence to ask for more.

TRYING TO MAKE IT BETTER

Recent changes in the way health services are organised have been made with the intention of getting rid of the 'postcode lottery' discussed in the previous chapter and making the way healthcare is provided fairer for everybody. Standards for the care everyone with kidney failure should expect from their doctors and nurses have been drawn up. We hope that they will help all patients to receive equally good care – and indeed to complain if they do not receive it.

THE RENAL NATIONAL SERVICE FRAMEWORK

In April 1998 the UK government launched a programme of National Service Frameworks. This was part of a number of measures that were introduced in the NHS Plan to raise quality and decrease variations in service in the NHS. These National Service Frameworks (or NSFs) cover a range of conditions including mental health, cancer and diabetes.

The idea behind the National Service Frameworks is that patients and their doctors should be the ones making choices about health. (All too often, it may appear that these choices are being made by policy makers.) The NSFs also stress the importance of giving local community services and GPs opportunities to improve health in their area.

The Renal National Service Framework (NSF) is in two parts. Part 1 was published in January 2004. It sets out five standards and identifies 30 markers of good practice which the NHS will need to deliver by 2014. These are aimed at helping the health services to manage demand, increase fairness of access – and improve choice and quality in dialysis and kidney transplant services. Part 2, which was published in 2005, focuses on the prevention of ERF, primary care, and end-of-life care.

The NSF was written and developed by a team of external reference groups (ERGs), which brought together health professionals, patients and carers, health service managers, partner agencies, and other advocates. The Department of Health was also involved in supporting the ERGs and managing the overall process.

The five standards set out in Part 1 are as follows:

Standard 1 – A patient-centred service

'All children, young people and adults with chronic kidney disease are to have access to information that enables them with their carers to make informed decisions and encourages partnership in decision making, with an agreed care plan that supports them in managing their condition to achieve the best possible quality of life.'

Standard 2 – Preparation and choice

'All children, young people and adults approaching established renal failure are to receive timely preparation for renal replacement therapy so the complications and progression of their disease are minimised, and their choice of clinically appropriate treatment options is maximised.'

Standard 3 – Elective dialysis access surgery

'All children, young people and adults with established

renal failure are to have timely and appropriate surgery for permanent vascular or peritoneal dialysis access, which is monitored and maintained to achieve its maximum longevity.'

Standard 4 – Dialysis
'Renal services are to ensure the delivery of high quality clinically appropriate forms of dialysis which are designed around individual needs and preferences and are available to patients of all ages throughout their lives.'

Standard 5 – Transplantation
'All children, young people and adults likely to benefit from a kidney transplant are to receive a high quality service which supports them in managing their transplant and enables them to achieve the best possible quality of life.'

Part 2 focuses on 'Quality requirements', as listed below:

Quality requirement 1: Prevention and early detection of chronic kidney disease
This quality requirement stresses the importance of identifying kidney failure early, especially where people are at a higher than average risk of developing kidney disease or having it undiagnosed. Early detection will give doctors the best possible chance of helping the person to manage his or her health in such a way that their kidney function will be preserved for as long as possible.

Quality requirement 2: Minimising the progression and consequences of chronic kidney disease
This stresses the importance of following up and monitoring the health of people with chronic kidney disease in order to reduce the risk of progression and complications.

Quality requirement 3: Acute renal failure
People at risk of, or suffering from, acute renal failure need to be identified promptly, with hospital services delivering high quality, clinically appropriate care in partnership with specialised renal teams.

Quality requirement 4: End-of-life care
People with established renal failure must be treated with honesty and respect and given appropriate information about the choices available to them. Plans for care in the period towards the end of life should be agreed by health professionals in consultation with the individuals themselves, so that any palliative care plan is built specifically around their own needs and preferences.

The NSF goes on to make the point that these standards and quality requirements apply to *all* people with, or at risk of, kidney failure. In some cases, for example, children and young people and some older people, the standards also apply (in varying degrees) to families, guardians or carers.

DELIVERING RENAL SERVICES
Traditionally services for people with ERF have been centred around hospital haemodialysis in a limited number of main renal units where renal consultants, inpatient and investigative facilities are based. In the 1970s and 1980s, programmes of home haemodialysis and peritoneal dialysis were established. The 1990s saw the development of a 'hub and spoke' model with many main renal units supported by one or more satellite haemodialysis units closer to patients' homes. In some cases the traditional hub and spoke model has evolved into a so-called 'clinical network', whereby the majority of renal care is as close to patients' homes as possible.

The renal NSF aims to help renal services to build

on the most successful elements of these models, while providing a more responsive service closer to home. More about the NSF for renal patients and what it might mean for you can be found on the Department of Health's website (see *page 161* for address details).

THE PATIENTS' ROLE IN ALL THIS

The Expert Patient Programme

The Expert Patient Programme is an NHS based patient-training programme that was set up in 2002. It is designed to help people to cope with long-term illnesses better by teaching them to look after themselves. To become an Expert Patient you need to attend a "Self-Management" course that will help you:

- Manage your medication
- Reduce levels of depression, fatigue and anxiety
- Improve communication with healthcare professionals such as specialist doctors and nurses
- Improve relaxation, exercise and diet
- Help you to be independent and more mobile
- Improve your job or voluntary work prospects
- Improve or maintain your quality of life

The course takes place over six weeks with one 2-hour session each week. So far the Expert Patient Programme has shown the following benefits:

- Fewer consultations
- Shorter waiting lists
- Fewer missed appointments
- Prescription cost savings

- Better communication with patients and healthcare providers
- Fewer admissions to hospital

To find out about The Expert Patient Programme in your area, visit www.expertpatients.nhs.uk

Patients' voices, patients' rights

With the publication of the Renal NSF came a great opportunity for patients and relatives or carers to become involved in improving the provision of renal services. Where NSF standards are not being met (and there is a shortfall in available treatment), or where patients feel they are not getting the choices they deserve, there are some things they can do about it. If you, or someone you care about, is in this position here are some suggestions:

- Become involved in your local renal network.
- If you feel that local services are not up to standard, why not write to your local newspaper? Publicity is a powerful tool.
- Join your local Kidney Patients' Association if there is one. If there is not one, consider whether you might be the person to start one.
- It is also a good idea to join the National Kidney Federation (NKF) which speaks for all kidney patients and has links with the All-Party Parliamentary Group for Kidneys (APPGK) – a group of MPs who fight for resources for kidney patients.
- Another national charity, the British Kidney Patient Association (BKPA) also provides information.
- Write to your MP or, even better; visit his or her local surgery. Not all politicians are aware of the major problems in British kidney medicine.

Whether you do one or all of these, keep at it!

KEY FACTS

1 There is simply not enough care for patients with kidney disease throughout the UK. A major reason for this is inadequate funding which makes providing and staffing a renal unit very difficult.

2 The amount and type of dialysis provided around the country varies significantly.

3 There is a shortage, of kidneys for transplant. More kidneys from living donors are needed to reduce the shortfall and relatives, partners and friends could consider donating a kidney to a loved one.

4 There is more information available, allowing patients to make choices, with regards to their care. It is debatable whether the choices are real.

5 A National Service Framework (NSF) for the care of renal patients has been developed. The aim of this is to give responsibility for care back to patients and their doctors.

6 Part 1 gives 5 standards and 30 markers of good practice to ensure that services for dialysis and transplant patients are of an appropriate standard everywhere in the UK.

7 Part 2 of the renal NSF focuses on the prevention of established renal failure, primary care, and care at the end of life. It lists four quality requirements relevant to these areas.

8 The Expert Patient Programme enables patients to help themselves and each other.

9 Patients have a right to be heard. Joining relevant organisations and writing to the local paper or your MP is a good place to start.

10 The renal community is attempting to reduce carbon emissions to help the environment.

GLOSSARY

This glossary provides brief explanations of the various technical words and abbreviations used in this book. Words printed in *italic* type have their own glossary entry.

Abdomen The lower part of the trunk, below the chest. Commonly called the tummy or belly.

Access A method of gaining entry to the bloodstream to allow *dialysis*. Access methods used for *haemodialysis* include *a catheter*, *fistula* or *graft*.

Acid A chemical that builds up in the blood in *kidney failure*.

Acute A word meaning short term and of rapid onset, usually requiring a rapid response.

Adequacy This term is used to describe the tests that are used to see how much *dialysis* a patient is getting. Samples of the *dialysis fluid*, blood and samples of *urine* are used to measure the dialysis adequacy.

Albumin A type of *protein* that occurs in the blood. Low blood levels may be linked to *malnutrition*.

Alfacalcidol A *vitamin D* supplement.

ALG Abbreviation for anti-lymphocyte globulin, a strong treatment against the *rejection* of a *transplant kidney*.

Alkali A substance that is the chemical opposite of an acid.

Alpha-blocker A type of *blood pressure* tablet – examples include doxazosin and terazosin.

Aluminium hydroxide A commonly-used type of *phosphate binder,* used to help prevent and treat *renal bone disease*. An example of aluminium hydroxide is Alu-Cap.

Amino acids Substances from which *proteins* are built up.

Anaemia A shortage of *red blood cells* in the body, causing tiredness, shortness of breath and pale skin. One of the functions of the *kidneys* is to make *erythropoietin*, which stimulates the *bone marrow* to make *blood cells*. In *kidney failure*, EPO is not made, and anaemia results.

Angiogram A type of X-ray that uses a special dye to show the *blood vessels*. The dye is put into the blood vessels via a tube that is inserted into the groin and passed up to the *kidneys*.

Angiotensin II (A2) antagonist A type of blood pressure tablet that can make kidney function worse, although it can be useful in certain situations. Also known as an ARB.

Angiotensin-converting enzyme (ACE) inhibitor A type of *blood pressure* tablet that can make kidney function worse, although it is useful in certain situations.

Ankle oedema An abnormal build-up of fluid in the skin around the ankles. It is an early sign of *fluid overload*.

Antibiotic drugs A group of drugs used to treat infections caused by *bacteria*.

Antibodies Substances that normally help the body to fight infection. They are made by *white blood cells*. After a *transplant*, antibodies can attack the new *kidney* and cause *rejection*.

Antibody incompatible transplantation A technique for increasing the likelihood of successful transplant between a donor and recipient who are not well matched. It involves using particularly strong immunsuppression combined with a dialysis-like process called plasmapharesis and other strong drugs.

Antigen A type of *protein* that occurs on the outer surface of all the cells in a person's body. Antigens act as a 'friendly face' for the cells. The *immune system* normally recognises the friendly face of the body's own *cells*, and does not attack or reject them.

APD Abbreviation for automated peritoneal dialysis. A form of *peritoneal dialysis* that uses a machine to drain the *dialysis fluid* out of the patient and replace it with fresh solution. APD is usually carried out overnight while the patient sleeps.

ARB another name for an *Angiotensin II (A2) antagonist*

Arteries *Blood vessels* that carry blood from the heart to the rest of the body.

Artificial kidney Another name for the *dialyser* or filtering unit of a *dialysis machine*.

ATG Abbreviation for anti-thymocyte globulin, a strong treatment against the *rejection* of a *transplant kidney*.

.

Dialysis machine The machine used to perform *haemodialysis*. It includes a *dialyser*, which filters the patient's blood. The machine helps to pump the patient's blood through the dialyser, and monitors the dialysis process as it takes place.

Dialysis membrane A thin layer of tissue or plastic with many tiny holes in it, through which the process of *dialysis* takes place. In *peritoneal dialysis*, the patient's *peritoneum* provides the dialysis membrane. For *haemodialysis*, the dialysis membrane is made of plastic. In each case, the membrane keeps the *dialysis fluid* separate from the blood (essential because dialysis fluid is toxic if it flows directly into the blood). However, the tiny holes in the membrane make it *semi-permeable*, allowing water and various substances to pass through it.

Diastolic blood pressure A *blood pressure* reading taken when the heart is relaxed. It is taken after the *systolic blood pressure*, and is the second figure in a blood pressure measurement. It should be 80 mmHg or less.

Diffusion A process by which substances pass from a stronger to a weaker solution. Diffusion is one of the key processes in *dialysis* (the other is *ultrafiltration*). During dialysis, body wastes such as *creatinine* pass from the blood into the *dialysis fluid*. At the same time, useful substances such as *bicarbonate* and *calcium* pass from the dialysis fluid into the blood.

Diuretic drugs The medical name for water tablets. These drugs increase the amount of *urine* that is passed. Two commonly used diuretics are *furosemide* and bumetanide.

Donor A person who donates (gives) an organ to another person (the recipient).

Donor kidney A *kidney* that has been donated.

Doppler scan A type of *ultrasound scan* (sound-wave picture) that provides information about blood flow through the *arteries*.

ECG Abbreviation for *electrocardiogram*.

ECHO Abbreviation for *echocardiogram*.

Echocardiogram (ECHO) A type of *ultrasound scan* (sound-wave picture) that shows how well the heart is working.

eGFR Estimated *glomerular filtration rate*. The term is generally applied to a test which measures how well the kidneys are working. It is normally around 100 mls/min, which approximates to 100 % of normal kidney function. It

is similar to the creatinine clearance test and is used mainly in the pre-dialysis period.

Electrocardiogram (ECG) A test that shows the electrical activity within the heart.

End-stage renal failure (ESRF) An alternative name for *established renal failure*.

End-stage renal disease (ESRD) An alternative name for *established renal failure*.

EPO Abbreviation for *erythropoietin*.

ERF Abbreviation for *established renal failure*.

Erythropoietin (EPO) A *hormone*, made by the *kidneys*, which stimulates the *bone marrow* to produce red blood cells.

Erythropoietin stimulating agent (ESA) A type of medication which stimulates the body's own production of erythropoietin *(EPO)*. ESAs are usually given by injection.

ESA Abbreviation for *erythropoietin stimulating agent*.

Established renal failure (ERF) A term for advanced chronic *kidney failure*. People who develop ERF will die within a few weeks unless treated by *dialysis* or *transplantation*. These treatments control ERF but cannot cure it. Once a patient has developed ERF, they will always have it, *even after a transplant*.

ESRF Abbreviation for *end-stage renal failure*.

ESRD Abbreviation for *end-stage renal disease*.

Exit site The point where a *catheter* comes out through the skin. Exit site infections can be a problem for *peritoneal dialysis* patients.

Ferritin A substance in the blood that indicates how much *iron* is present. The more iron there is in the body, the higher the level of ferritin in the blood.

Fistula An enlarged *vein*, usually at the wrist or elbow, that gives access to the bloodstream for *haemodialysis*. The fistula is created by a surgeon in a small operation. It is done by joining a vein to an *artery*. This increases the flow of blood through the vein and causes it to enlarge, making it suitable for haemodialysis needles.

FK506 Another name for *tacrolimus*.

Flucloxacillin An antibiotic used to treat *exit site* infections of *peritoneal dialysis* and *haemodialysis* catheters.

Fluid overload A condition in which the body contains too much water. It is caused by drinking too much fluid, or not losing enough. Fluid overload occurs in *kidney failure* because one of the main functions of the *kidneys* is to remove excess water. Fluid overload often occurs with high *blood pressure*. Excess fluid first gathers around the ankles (*ankle oedema*) and may later settle in the lungs (*pulmonary oedema*).

Furosemide A commonly used *diuretic*.

Gentamicin An antibiotic used to treat *peritonitis*.

GFR An abbreviation for glomerular filtration rate, also the name of a test which indicates how effectively the kidneys get rid of waste by measuring the number of millilitres of blood the kidneys are able to filter in one minute.

Glomerulonephritis Inflammation of the glomeruli, which is one of the causes of *kidney failure*.

Glomerulus One of the tiny filtering units inside the *kidney*.

Glucose A type of sugar. There is normally a small amount of glucose in the blood. This amount is not usually increased in people with *kidney failure* unless they also have *diabetes mellitus*. Glucose is the main substance in *peritoneal dialysis* fluid, drawing excess water into the *dialysis fluid* from the blood by *osmosis*.

Graft A type of access for *haemodialysis*. The graft is a small plastic tube that connects an *artery* to a *vein*. It is inserted into the arm or leg by a surgeon. *Haemodialysis* needles are inserted into the graft, which can be used many hundreds of times.

Haemodialysis A form of *dialysis* in which the blood is cleaned outside the body, in a machine called a *dialysis machine* or *kidney machine*. The machine contains a filter called the dialyser or artificial kidney. Each dialysis session lasts for 3–5 hours, and sessions are usually needed 2–3 times a week.

Haemodialysis catheter A plastic tube used to gain access to the bloodstream for *haemodialysis*.

Haemodialysis unit The part of a hospital where patients go for *haemodialysis*.

Haemoglobin (Hb) A substance in red blood cells that carries oxygen around the body. Blood levels of haemoglobin are measured to look for *anaemia*. A low Hb level indicates anaemia.

Hb Abbreviation for *haemoglobin*.

Hepatitis An infection of the liver, usually caused by a *virus*. Two main types, called hepatitis B and hepatitis C, can be passed on by blood contact. This means that *dialysis*

patients, especially those on *haemodialysis*, have an increased risk of getting these infections. Care is taken to reduce this risk, and regular virus checks are made on all kidney patients.

HIV Human immunodeficiency virus, the virus that causes AIDS. Tests for this virus are carried out before a patient can have a *transplant*. This is because HIV may be present and inactive in the patient's body but can be activated by the transplant and *immuno-suppressant drugs*.

Home haemodialysis Treatment on a *dialysis machine* installed in a patient's own home. For home haemodialysis to be considered, the patient must have a partner or friend who is able to supervise every *dialysis* session.

Hormones Substances that act as chemical messengers in the body. They are produced in parts of the body called endocrine glands. Hormones travel around the body in the blood, and control how other parts of the body work. For example, *parathyroid hormone* from the *parathyroid glands* in the neck affects *kidney* function.

HTA Abbreviation for Human Tissue Authority. This government body must give approval to all *living donor transplants*.

Hyperparathyroidism A disorder in which the *parathyroid glands* make too much *parathyroid hormone*.

Immune system The body's natural defence system. It includes organs (such as the spleen and appendix), lymph nodes (including the 'glands' in the neck) and specialist *white blood cells* called *lymphocytes*. The immune system protects the body from infections, foreign bodies and cancer. To prevent *rejection* of a *transplant kidney*, it is necessary for patients to take *immuno-suppressant drugs*.

Immuno-suppressant drugs A group of drugs used to dampen down the *immune system* to prevent *rejection* of a *transplant kidney*. Commonly used examples are *ciclosporin*, *azathioprine*, *prednisolone*, *tacrolimus* and *mycophenolate mofetil*.

Intravenous pyelogram (IVP) A special X-ray of the *kidneys*. A dye that shows up on X-rays is used to show the drainage system of the kidneys. The dye is injected into the patient's arm, travels in the blood to the kidneys, and is passed from the body in the *urine*.

Iron A substance that is necessary to prevent *anaemia*. A low blood *ferritin* indicates low levels of iron in the body.

failure, phosphate tends to build up in the blood. High phosphate levels occur with low calcium levels in people with *renal bone disease*.

Phosphate binders Tablets that help prevent a build-up of *phosphate* in the body. Phosphate binders combine with phosphate in food so that it passes it out of the body in the faeces. The most commonly used phosphate binders are *calcium carbonate* and *aluminium hydroxide*.

Plasma The liquid part of the blood in which the blood *cells* float.

Platelets A type of blood *cell* that helps the blood to clot.

Polycystic kidney disease (PCKD) An inherited disease (a disease that runs in families) in which both kidneys are full ('poly' means 'many') of cysts (abnormal fluid-filled lumps). PCKD is one of the causes of *kidney failure*. It is diagnosed by an *ultrasound scan*.

Potassium A mineral that is normally present in the blood, and which is measured in the *biochemistry blood test*. Either too much or too little potassium can be dangerous, causing the heart to stop. People with *kidney failure* may need to restrict the amount of potassium in their diet.

Prednisolone A drug used to prevent or treat the *rejection* of a *transplant kidney*.

Proteins Chemical components of the body, formed from *amino acids*. The body needs supplies of protein in the diet to build muscles and to repair itself.

PTH Abbreviation for *parathyroid hormone*.

Pulmonary oedema A serious condition in which fluid builds up in the lungs, causing breathlessness. People with *kidney failure* develop pulmonary oedema if *fluid overload* is not treated promptly.

Pyelonephritis Inflammation of the drainage system of the *kidneys*, one of the causes of *kidney failure*. It can be diagnosed by an ultrasound scan, an intravenous pyelogram or a nuclear medicine scan.

Radio-isotope scan A method of obtaining pictures of the body's interior, also called a *radio-nuclide scan* or *nuclear medicine scan*. A small amount of a mildly radioactive substance is either swallowed or injected into the bloodstream. The substance gathers in certain parts of the body, which then show up on pictures taken by a special machine.

Radio-nuclide scan Another name for a *radio-isotope scan*.

Recipient In the context of *transplantation*, a person who receives an organ from another person (the donor).

Red blood cells *Cells* in the blood which carry oxygen from the lungs around the body.

Reflux The movement of a liquid, such as *urine*, in the opposite direction to normal. The word 'reflux' is sometimes used to mean *reflux nephropathy*.

Reflux nephropathy A condition in which *urine* passes back up from the *bladder*, through the *ureters*, to the *kidneys*, where it can cause infections. It occurs because a valve that normally prevents the backflow of urine from the bladder is faulty. Reflux nephropathy is one of the causes of *kidney failure*.

Rejection The process by which a patient's *immune system* recognises a *transplant kidney* (or other transplanted organ) as not its 'own', and then tries to destroy it and remove it from the body. Rejection can be *acute* or *chronic*.

Renal Adjective meaning relating to the *kidneys*.

Renal bone disease A complication of *kidney failure*, in which bone health is affected by abnormally low blood levels of *calcium* and *vitamin D*, and high levels of *phosphate*. Without treatment, renal bone disease can result in bone pain and fractures.

Renal unit A hospital department that treats disorders of the *kidneys*.

Renovascular disease Atheroma affecting the *blood vessels* that supply the kidneys ('reno' means relating to the kidney, and 'vascular' means relating to the blood vessels). Renovascular disease is a common cause of *kidney failure* in older patients.

Residual renal function (RRF) The amount of kidney function that a patient on dialysis has. This varies from patient to patient. It is likely the RRF will reduce over a period of time, and in many patients, it eventually disappears altogether. A *creatinine clearance test* is used to assess RRF.

Rifampicin An *antibiotic drug* used to treat long-term *exit site* infections of *peritoneal dialysis* catheters.

Rigors Cold shivers that sometimes occur with a fever. They can be a symptom of an infected *haemodialysis catheter*.

RRF Abbreviation for *residual renal function*.

Satellite haemodialysis unit A place where some patients go for *haemodialysis* away from the main hospital *renal unit*. Satellite units have relatively few nurses, and are suitable only for healthy patients, who do some of the haemodialysis preparation themselves. These units tend to be more easily accessible to patients than most main hospital buildings.

Scan One of several techniques for obtaining pictures of the body's interior without using conventional X-rays. Examples include *CT scans*, *MRI scans*, *radio-isotope scans* and *ultrasound scans*.

Semi-permeable An adjective, often used to describe a *membrane*, meaning that it will allow some but not all substances to pass through it. Substances with smaller *molecules* will pass through the holes in the membrane, whereas substances with larger molecules will not.

Sirolimus A new immuno-suppressant drug which is an alternative to ciclosporin or tacrolimus.

Sodium A mineral that is normally present in the blood, and which is measured in the *biochemistry blood test*. Sodium levels are not usually a problem for people with *kidney failure* and are quite easily controlled by *dialysis*.

Sphygmomanometer The instrument used to measure *blood pressure*.

Staphylococcus One of a group of *bacteria* responsible for various infections (often called 'staph' infections). A common cause of *peritonitis* in patients on *peritoneal dialysis*, and of *line infections* in *haemodialysis* patients.

Statins A group of drugs that reduce lipid levels in the blood, especially cholesterol. Examples include atorvastatin and simvastatin.

Systolic blood pressure A *blood pressure* reading taken when the heart squeezes as it beats. The systolic blood pressure is measured before the *diastolic blood pressure* and is the first figure in a blood pressure measurement.

Tacrolimus An *immuno-suppressant drug*, also known as FK506, which is an alternative to *ciclosporin*.

Tissue A collection of similar *cells* that share a similar function, such as skin cells or *kidney cells*.

Tissue type A set of inherited characteristics on the surface of *cells*. Each person's tissue type has six components (three from each parent). Although there are only three main sorts of tissue type characteristic (called A, B and DR), each of these comes in 20 or more different versions. Given the large number of possibilities, it is unusual for there to be an exact tissue type match between a *transplant kidney* and its recipient. However, the more characteristics that match, the more likely a *transplant* is to succeed.

Tissue typing A blood test that identifies a person's *tissue type*.

Toxins Poisons. One of the main functions of the *kidneys* is to remove toxins from the blood (a process known as *clearance*).

Transplant A term used to mean either a *transplant kidney* (or other transplant organ) or a *transplant operation*.

Transplantation The replacement of an organ in the body by another person's organ. Many different organs can now be successfully transplanted, including the *kidneys*, liver, bowel, heart, lungs, pancreas, skin and bones.

Transplant kidney A *kidney* removed from one person (the donor) and given to another person (the recipient). Transplant kidneys may be either *deceased donor transplants*, *living related transplants* or *living unrelated transplants*.

Transplant operation The surgical operation by which a patient is given a donated organ. The operation to insert a *transplant kidney* takes about 2–3 hours. The new *kidney* is placed lower in the *abdomen* than the patient's own kidneys, which are usually left in place. *Blood vessels* attached to the transplant kidney are connected to the patient's blood supply, and the new kidney's *ureter* is connected to the patient's *bladder*.

Transplant waiting list A system that seeks to find the 'right' transplant organ for the 'right' patient. It is co-ordinated nationally by *UKT*, whose computer compares patients' details (including *blood group* and *tissue type*) with those of deceased donor organs that become available. The average waiting time for a *deceased donor transplant kidney* is about 2 years.

Tuberculosis A bacterium that can cause long-term infections. It is an unusual source of PD peritonitis.

Tunnel infection A possible problem for patients on *peritoneal dialysis* (PD). It occurs when an infection spreads from the *exit site* into the 'tunnel' (i.e. the route of the PD catheter through the abdominal wall).

Ultrafiltration The removal of excess water from the body. Ultrafiltration is one of the two main functions of the

USEFUL ADDRESSES AND WEBSITES

Addresses correct at time of going to press, but please note that all are subject to change from time to time.

Action on Smoking and Health (ASH)
102 Clifton Street
London EC2A 4HW
Tel: 020 7739 5902
Fax: 020 7613 0531
Helpline: 0800 169 0169
Website: www.ash.org.uk
Information on how smoking affects medical conditions.

Age UK
FREEPOST
London N1 9BR
Tel: 0800 107 8977
Website: www.ageuk.org
A new organisation combining Age Concern and Help the Aged. The Age UK family also includes Age Cymru, Age NI and Age Scotland. Provides advice and publications on a range of subjects for older people.

Assist UK
Redbank House
4 St Chad's Street
Manchester M8 8QA
Tel: 0870 770 2866
Textphone: 0870 770 5813
Website: www.assist-uk.org
Coordinates the work of Disabled Living Centres in the UK. Can provide details of centres where you can try out furniture, aids and equipment designed to help people who are older or have disabilities.

British Association of Counselling
BACP House
35–37 Albert Street
Rugby
Warwickshire CV21 2SG
Tel: 08788 550 899
Website: www.counselling.co.uk
Send s.a.e. for information about counselling services in your area, and publications list.

British Heart Foundation
1 Fitzhardinge Street
London W1H 6DH
Helpline: 0845 070 8070
Website: www.bhf.org.uk
Funds research, promotes education and raises money for equipment to treat people with heart disease.

British Kidney Patient Association
Bordon
Hampshire GU35 9JZ
Tel: 01420 472 021
Fax: 01420 4725 831
Website: www.britishkidney-pa.co.uk
Provides information and advice to people with kidney illnesses throughout the UK. Grants available.

British Organ and Donation Society (BODY)
Balsham
Cambridge CB21 4DL
Tel: 01223 893636
Email: body@argonet.co.uk
Website: body.orpheusweb.co.uk
Provides information on transplant and donation.

Cancerlink
Macmillan Cancer Relief
89 Albert Embankment
London SE1 7UQ
Tel: 020 7840 7840
Fax: 020 7840 7841
Helpline: 0808 808 0000
Website: www.cancerlink.org
Helps cancer patients, families and carers with practical and emotional support.

Carers UK
20 Great Dover Street
London SE1 4LX
Tel: 020 7378 4999
Fax: 020 7378 9871
Advice line: 0808 808 7777
Website: www.carersonline.org.uk
Offers information and support to all people who have to care for others due to medical or other problems.

Citizens Advice
Myddleton House
115–123 Pentonville Road
London N1 9LZ
Tel: 020 7833 2181 (admin only; no advice available on this number)
Head office of a national charity offering a wide variety of practical, legal and financial advice through its network of local branches throughout the UK and its Adviceguide website.

Crossroads – Caring for Carers
10 Regent Place
Rugby
Warwicks CV21 2PN
Tel: 01788 573653
Helpline: 0845 450 0350
Website: www.crossroads.org.uk
Supports and delivers high quality services (including respite care) for carers and people in need via its local branches.

Crossroads Scotland Care Attendant Schemes
24 George Square
Glasgow G2 1EG
Tel: 0141 226 3793
Fax: 0141 221 7130
Website:
www.crossroads.scotland.co.uk
Provides a paid, trained person to offer respite care in the home.

CRUSE – Bereavement Care
126 Sheen Road
Richmond
Surrey TW9 1UR
Tel: 020 8940 4818
Fax: 020 8940 7638
Helpline: 0870 167 1677
Website:
www.crusebereavementcare.org.uk
Offers information and practical advice. Sells literature and has local branches that provide one-to-one counselling to people who have been bereaved. Runs training in bereavement counselling for professionals.

Department for Work and Pensions
Helpline: 0800 137 177
Government information service offering advice on benefits for people with disabilities, and their carers.

Department of Health
Richmond House
79 Whitehall
London SW1A 2NS
Website: www.dh.gov.uk

Depression Alliance
212 Spitfire Studios
63–71 Collier Street
London N1 9BE
Tel: 0845 123 2320
Website:
www.depressionalliance.org.uk
Offers support and understanding to anyone affected by depression, and relatives who want help. Has a network of self help groups, correspondence schemes and a range of literature. Send s.a.e. for information.

Diabetes UK
10 Parkway
London NW1 7AA
Tel: 020 7424 1000
Fax: 020 7424 1000
Helpline: 0845 120 29 60
Website: www.diabetes.org.uk
Provides advice and information for people with diabetes and their families; has local support groups.

Kidney Research UK
King's Chambers
Priestgate
Peterborough PE1 1FG
Tel: 0845 070 7601
Helpline: 0845 300 14 99
Email: info@ kidneyresearchuk.org
Website: www.kidneyresearchuk.org
Funds research into kidney disease, its causes and treatment. Works to raise awareness of kidney disease.

Medic-Alert Foundation
1 Bridge Wharf
156 Caledonian Road
London N1 9UU
Tel: 020 7833 3034
Fax: 020 2213 5653
e-mail: info@medicalert.co.uk
Offers a selection of jewellery with internationally recognised medical symbol: 24 hour emergency phoneline.

MIND (National Association for Mental Health)
15-19 Broadway
Stratford
London E15 4BQ
Tel: 020 8519 2122
Helpline: 0845 766 0163
Website: www.mind.org.uk
Mental health organisation working for a better life for everyone experiencing mental distress. Has information and offers support via local branches.

National Kidney Federation
The Point
Coach Road
Shireoaks
Worksop
Notts S81 8BW
Helpline: 0845 601 02 09
Email: nkf@kidney.org.uk
Website: www.kidney.org.uk
Aims to promote, throughout the United Kingdom, the welfare of people suffering from kidney disease or renal failure, and those relatives and friends who care for them.

NHS Direct
England and Wales: 0845 4647
Website: www.nhsdirect.nhs.uk
Speak to a nurse for some commonsense advice about your health.

NHS 24
Scotland: 0845 424 24 24
Website: www.nhsdirect.nhs.uk
NHS Direct for Scotland.

NHS Blood and Transplant
Organ Donation and Transplant Directorate
Fox Den Road
Stoke Gifford
Bristol BS34 8RR
Tel: 0117 975 7575
Fax: 0117 975 7577
Website: www.organdonation.nhs.uk
Provides information about donating organs and how patients can benefit from organ donation.

National Institute for Health and Clinical Excellence (NICE)
Website: www.nice.org.uk
The organisation responsible for providing national guidance on drugs and treatments offered in the NHS.

Outsiders
45 Leroy House
435 Essex Road
London N1 3QP
Tel: 020 7354 8291
Website: www.outsiders.org.uk
A national self-help organisation that provides advice about sexual relationships to people with diabilities.

Patients Association
PO Box 935
Harrow
Middlesex HA1 3YJ
Tel: 020 8423 9111
Fax: 020 8423 9119
Helpline: 0845 608 44 55
Website: www.patients-association.com
Provides advice on patients' rights.

RADAR (Royal Association for Disability and Rehabilitation)
12 City Forum
250 City Road
London EC1V 8AF
Tel: 020 7250 3222
Fax: 020 7250 0212
Website: www.radar.org.uk
Campaigns to improve the rights and care of people with a disability. Sells special key to access locked public toilets for the disabled.

Registered Nursing Homes Association
15 Highfield Road
Edgbaston
Birmingham B15 3DU
Tel: 0121 454 2511
Fax: 0121 454 9032
Website: www.rnha.co.uk
Information about registered nursing homes in your area that meet the standards set by the Association.

Relate
Premier House
Carolina Court
Lakeside
Doncaster DN4 5RA
Tel: 0300 100 1234
(or see your phonebook for local branch)
Website: www.relate.org.uk
Offers relationship counselling via local branches, and publishes information on health, sexual, self-esteem, depression, bereavement and remarriage issues.

Renal Patient View
Website: www.renalpatientview.org
This site is currently available through selected renal units only, but in time it will enable all patients to view their own results and care pathways on the Internet.

Renal Registry of the United Kingdom Southmead Hospital
Southmead Road
Bristol BS10 5NB
Tel: 0117 959 5665
Fax: 0117 959 5664
Website: www.renalreg.com
Collects, analyses and presents data about the incidence, clinical management and outcome of renal disease.

Sexual Dysfunction Association
Windmill Place Business Centre
2–4 Windmill Lane
Southall UB2 4NU
Helpline: 0870 774 35 71
Website: www.sda.uk.net
Association providing help and advice on sexual and relationship problems.

United Kingdom Register of Counsellors
P O Box 1050
Rugby
Warwickshire CV21 2HZ
Tel: 0870 443 5232
Fax: 0870 443 5161
Part of British Association of Counselling and Psychotherapy Regulatory body which provides details of registered counsellors who offer safe and accountable practice.

Vitalise
12 City Forum
250 City Road
London EC1V 8AF
Tel: 0845 345 1972
Fax: 0845 345 1978
Website: www.vitalise.org.uk
Formerly known as the Winged Fellowship Trust, provides holidays and respite care for disabled people and their carers.

INDEX

Page numbers followed by italic *g* refer to glossary items

importance of 75
food 108
hyperkalaemia (excess potassium) 74
hyperparathyroidism 153g

I

Icodextrin 62
IgA nephropathy 78
immune system 79, 97, 153g
suppression *see* immuno-suppressant drugs
immuno-suppressant drugs 94, 99, 153g
cancer and 101–2, 131
delaying dialysis 9
side effects 100–101
impotence *see* erectile dysfunction
independence
and peritoneal dialysis 63
infection
deaths from 135
exit site 65
and haemodialysis 72, 75–6
line 75–6
peritonitis 65
after transplant 101
tunnel 65
information 143–4
seeking 114
insulin 44, 100
Intensive Care Units (ICUs) 141
intravenous drip 94–5
intravenous pyelogram (IVP) 6, 48, 153g
intravenous urogram (IVU) 48
irbesartan 28
iron 153g
blood test *see* ferritin
deficiency 33
tablets and injections 33, 46
irritability 30
isotope GFR (glomerular filtration rate) 49
itching 5, 36

IVP (intravenous pyelogram) 6, 48, 154g
IVU (intravenous urogram) 48

J

jaundice 45
joints, problems with 100
jugular line 71

K

kidney(s) 1, 3, 154g
artificial *see* dialyser (artificial kidney)
functions *see* kidney functions
location 1, 2
'small' 7
structure 3
kidney (renal) biopsy 6, 46–8, 154g
and rejection 98–9
kidney disease, chronic, NSF quality requirements 145
kidney donors 154g
see also donor(s)
kidney failure 4, 154g
acute 4
causes 5–7
causes of death 134–5
chronic 1, 4, 7, 145
death from 128
diagnosis 5
international comparisons 135–7
key facts 11
number of UK patients with 1
progression of 7, 8
signs of 8
stages of 8
survival chances 133–4
symptoms 5, 7, 8
treatment *see* treatments for kidney failure
see also established renal failure
kidney functions
blood pressure control 4
excess water removal 2, 3–4
keeping bones healthy 4

red blood cell manufacture 4
urine production 1–2
waste removal 2–3, 12
kidney machine 154g
see also dialysis (kidney) machine
kidney transplants 154g
benefits 77
number of 140–42
see also transplant(s); transplant kidney; transplant operation; transplantation
kidney units *see* renal units

L

labetalol 28
lactate 43
legs
cramps 5
restless 5
LFTs (liver function tests) 154g
life expectancy 133
lifestyle changes 113
haemodialysis 73
with peritoneal dialysis 63–4
line infection 75, 154g
lipids 154g
lisinopril 27
liver, urea production 12
liver function tests (LFTs) 45, 47, 154g
living donor transplants 85, 154g
benefits 85–6
choice of donor 88
compared with deceased donor transplants 86, 95
key facts 93
number of 141–3
patient survival after 86
preparation for 91
rejection risk 92
removal of kidney 91
risks 86
risks to donor 92
risks to recipient 92
tests for donors 88–9

The *Class Health* Feedback Form

We hope that you found this *Class Health* book helpful. We always appreciate readers' opinions and would be grateful if you could take a few minutes to complete this form for us.

❶ How did you acquire your copy of this book?

From my local library ☐

Read an article in a newspaper/magazine ☐

Found it by chance ☐

Recommended by a friend ☐

Recommended by a patient organisation/charity ☐

Recommended by a doctor/nurse/adviser ☐

Saw an advertisement ☐

❷ How much of the book have you read?

All of it ☐

More than half of it ☐

Less than half of it ☐

❸ Which copies/chapters have been most helpful?

....
....
....

❹ Overall, how useful to you was this *Class Health* book?

Extremely useful ☐

Very useful ☐

Useful ☐

❺ What did you find most helpful?

....
....
....

❻ What did you find least helpful?

....
....
....

❼ What did you find least helpful?

....
....
....

❽ Have you read any other health books?

Yes ☐   No ☐

If yes, which subjects did they cover?

....
....

How did this *Class Health* book compare?

Much better ☐

Better ☐

About the same ☐

Not as good ☐

❾ Would you recommend this book to a friend?

Yes ☐   No ☐

Thank you for your help. Please send your completed form to:

Class Publishing, FREEPOST, London W6 7BR

Surname .... First name ....

Title: Prof/Dr/Mr/Mrs/Ms ....

Address ....

....

Town .... Postcode ....

Country ....

☐ Please add my name and address to receive details of related books

[Please note, we will not pass on your details to any other company]

Have you found **Kidney Failure Explained** useful and practical? If so, you may be interested in other books from Class Publishing.

Eating Well for Kidney Health

Helena Jackson, Claire Green and Gavin James £17.99
This book is about good food, good drink and good health. It is full of simple, quick and great-tasting recipes for people with chronic kidney disease (CKD), along with their friends and families.

'Food is a joy, restrictions can be tiresome. This book shows you how to bypass tiresome and eat well.'
Timothy F Statham OBE, Chief Executive, National Kidney Federation

Eating Well with Kidney Failure

Helena Jackson, Annie Cassidy and Gavin James £17.99
If you have kidney failure, you need to adapt and change what you eat. But, as this practical and exciting new book shows, you don't need to go on a crash diet, or to deny yourself the foods you love – you just need to adapt your favourite recipes with kidney-friendly foods.

The authors have provided more than fifty delicious recipes to show you how this works in practice. The recipes have been analysed for their nutritional content and are coded to help you choose the most appropriate dishes for your individual requirements.

Living Well with Kidney Failure

Juliet Auer £14.99
This practical and inspiring book highlights the experiences of a number of very different people, from all walks of life, ages and family situations. These shared personal accounts celebrate the fullness of life that people living with kidney failure can, and do, achieve.

'This cheerful book will be a great help and encouragement to patients and their families trying to become experts on renal failure.' *Dr Christopher Winearls, Clinical Director of the Oxford Kidney Unit*

Kidney Dialysis and Transplants: Answers at your fingertips

Dr Andy Stein, Dr Rob Higgins and Janet Wild £14.99
This practical handbook for anyone with long-term kidney failure, and their families, contains practical, medically informed answers to over 430 questions asked by people with established renal failure.

'A first class book on kidney dialysis and transplants that is simple and accurate, and can be used to equal advantage by doctors and their patients.'
Dr Thomas Stuttaford, The Times

Kidney Transplants Explained

Dr Andy Stein, Dr Rob Higgins and Janet Wild £17.99
A successful kidney transplant can transform the life of a person with kidney failure, and people with a well functioning transplant often feel much fitter than they did on dialysis. However, it is essential to be thoroughly prepared for a kidney transplant. This book will help by answering all the questions about transplants and what they involve. Indispensable to people considering having a transplant or already living with one, this guide will also be valuable to anyone thinking about donating a kidney.

Type 1 Diabetes: Answers at your fingertips
Type 2 Diabetes: Answers at your fingertips

Dr Charles Fox and Dr Anne Kilvert Each £14.99

Our bestselling reference guide on diabetes has now been split into two books covering the two distinct forms of the disease. These books maintain the popular question and answer format to provide practical advice on every aspect of living with the condition.

'I have no hesitation in commending this book.' *Sir Steve Redgrave, Vice President, Diabetes UK*

PRIORITY ORDER FORM

Cut out or photocopy this form and send it (*post free in the UK*) to:

Class Publishing Priority Service
FREEPOST 16705
Macmillan Distribution
Basingstoke, RG21 6ZZ

Tel: 01256 302 699
Fax: 01256 812 558

Please send me urgently
(tick below)

*Post included price
per copy (UK only)*

☐	**Kidney Failure Explained**	£20.99
	(ISBN: 978 1 85959 236 6)	
☐	**Eating Well for Kidney Health**	£20.99
	(ISBN: 978 1 85959 204 5)	
☐	**Eating Well with Kidney Failure**	£20.99
	(ISBN: 978 1 85959 116 1)	
☐	**Living Well with Kidney Failure**	£17.99
	(ISBN: 978 185959 112 3)	
☐	**Kidney Dialysis and Transplants: Answers at your fingertips**	£17.99
	(ISBN: 978 185959 046 1)	
☐	**Kidney Transplants Explained**	£20.99
	(ISBN: 978 1 85959 193 2)	
☐	**Type 1 Diabetes: Answers at your fingertips**	£17.99
	(ISBN: 978 185959 175 8)	
☐	**Type 2 Diabetes: Answers at your fingertips**	£17.99
	(ISBN: 978 185959 176 5)	TOTAL _____

Easy ways to pay

Cheque: I enclose a cheque payable to Class Publishing for £ _____

Credit card: please debit my   ☐ Mastercard   ☐ Visa   ☐ Amex

Number _____ Expiry date _____

Name _____

My address for delivery is _____

_____

Town _____ County _____ Postcode _____

Telephone number (in case of query) _____

Credit card billing address if different from above _____

Class Publishing's guarantee: remember that if, for any reason, you are not satisfied with these books, we will refund all your money, without any questions asked. Prices and VAT rates may be altered for reasons beyond our control.